HeartSong

*Discover the Secret
to a Fulfilling Love Relationship*

**Conversations About
Love, Joy and Sex**

Also by Colin Hillstrom

YOUR 2ND LIFE
How to Live the Life You Always Wanted
* CD and Manual *

WHEN A MAN REALLY LOVES A WOMAN
Why We Must Love More
And What To Do About It

Also by Ariole K. Alei

BIRDS' EYE VIEW
A Travel Guide to the Universe

AWAKENING INSTINCT
The True Feminine Principle

♥

RUNNING THE GAUNTLET
Navigating Our Way to our Fully Embodied Potential

♥

WINDOWS THROUGH TIME
A 'Possible Evolution' Story
* A Trilogy *

ASCENSION TEACHINGS
The Original Memory
* Audio Cassette Series *

HeartSong

Discover the Secret
to a Fulfilling Love Relationship

Conversations About
Love, Joy and Sex

Colin Hillstrom
and
Ariole K. Alei

♥ HeartSong Solutions™

Vancouver, Canada

HeartSong Solutions™
Publish47- 2768 West Broadway
PO Ber, BC, Canada, V6K 4P4
Vaver-axis.net, www.HeartSongSolutions.ca
wy

ver Design: Jan Rosgen (www.janrosgen.com)
Justration: Jan Rosgen with Colin Hillstrom and Ariole K. Alei
Design and Layout: Ariole K. Alei
Editorial: Ariole K. Alei, Colin Hillstrom, MaryAnn Hager, Jan Rosgen,
Jan Henrikson and other kind souls
Production and Printing: Lulu, Inc.

Library and Archives Canada Cataloguing in Publication

Hillstrom, Colin, 1959
   HeartSong : discover the secret to a fulfilling relationship :
   conversations about love, joy and sex / Colin Hillstrom and Ariole
   K. Alei.

Includes bibliographical references.
ISBN-13 978-1-4116-9155-1
ISBN-10 1-4116-9155-5

   1. Love. 2. Interpersonal relations. I. Title.

HQ801.H449 2006 158.2 C2006-903838-4

Distribution: info@veraxis.net
     www.lulu.com/HeartSong

This 'conversation'
is dedicated
to all that has assisted us to learn –
people, creatures, nature, and life itself –
and to all those
journeying towards
loving, mature, respectful, joyous relationships …

Thank You

Contents

Acknowledgments

Throughout our lives we have met, journeyed with, and learned from so many people.

Special thanks to our parents Edith and Erich Mocek and Dorcas and Ray Wehner. To Colin's children Alex, Stefon, and Dominnik. To Ariole's siblings, their spouses, and offspring Tim and Ursula, Alastair and Emma, Jan, Claire, and Dave. To our many friends, teachers, and clients.

Special thanks also to Jan Rosgen for her cover design and illustrations which grace these pages.

And to you ... for sharing this journey of transformation and discovery with us.

Thank you!

Introduction

HeartSong - Discover the Secret to a Fulfilling Love Relationship - Conversations About Love, Joy and Sex is a transcribed conversation between Colin Hillstrom and Ariole K. Alei, Co-Founders of *Veraxis* Coaching and Training™ and **HeartSong Singles, Couples, Families, and Teens**. Colin and Ariole have lived and worked together for seven years. They have both been passionately involved in bringing out the best in themselves and others for several decades.

Life Balance

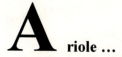 **A** riole …

Over the last few years we have worked with thousands of clients. What are some of the things that you've noticed, Colin, about people's relationships?

Colin …

Sadly, most people seem to suffer from a serious love deficiency. The majority over the age of 55 or 60 are either divorced, widowed or in bad relationships. Many younger people choose to be single because they are afraid or hesitant to be in a relationship. Many people in their mid thirties are stuck in marriages that have gone downhill within one or two years of their wedding. I talk to many people in their 60's and 70's who are deeply concerned about the well-being of their middle-aged children because they have become single parents or because they are in highly stressed relationships.

Ariole …

Do you ever see clients who are happily married?

Colin …

Unfortunately, very seldom. Mind you most people come to me because they need relationship help. But what I find out quickly is that they themselves know very few people - if anyone - who enjoys a healthy love relationship. Few people seem to have received good modeling from their parents about love, joy, sex and mutual respect. It isn't really a surprise then that people have become cynical about man / woman relationships.

Ariole …

So what do you discuss with these people?

Colin …

I speak with them about various approaches to life fulfillment, some of which I'm going to explain. For example, I talk to people about life balance. I talk to them about the blueprint of the human mind. We discuss stress and how to respond to it, amongst other topics.

Ariole …

Let's clarify what we mean by life balance and why it's so important to relationships.

Colin ...

Sure. Talking with someone about life balance helps them understand that their relationship is only one aspect of their whole life. For example, in addition to a significant other / marriage relationship, one also has to deal with career, money, health, family, friends, recreation, spiritual or personal growth, and last but not least, the quality of one's home environment. Much too often people focus or over-focus on one or two areas of their life and neglect all the others, thereby creating an imbalance which in itself causes stress and disharmony.

Ariole ...

Can you give an example of life balance?

Colin ...

Sure. Take a fifty-two year old male business owner who works sixty-five to seventy hours a week and hardly spends any quality time with his wife and children. He's also too exhausted to engage in meaningful recreational pursuits. To make things worse, he doesn't find time to eat well. What would this person's life balance be like? The point is, until someone addresses the reason why they're over-working themselves, they will most likely continue the same pattern in any relationship. The problem in that person's life is therefore not necessarily his bad relationship with his wife, but the fact that he's not taking a balanced approach to managing his life. It may just be a matter of time before he crashes. The number of men and women who are suffering from 'heart disease' is alarming …

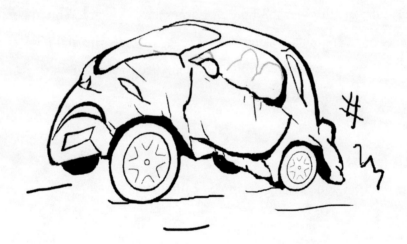

Ariole …

So if this person were to sit in front of you, how would you begin the process of Coaching him towards more fulfillment in his relationship?

Colin ...

I would speak to this person about 'his life', meaning that 'I have a life, this is my life, and therefore I am not my life.' Just like 'I have a car, therefore I am not my car. I am responsible for that which is mine, therefore I am also responsible for my life. My life is something that I can put in front of me. I can look at it. I can assess what needs to be done. And I can begin working on it.' In this way I help my client get a new context of his life, showing him how he can take responsible, positive action. Now that he sees that this is within his power, he regains hope. And all that I have to do is guide him to make meaningful commitments towards enhanced life balance so that he may enjoy his journey.

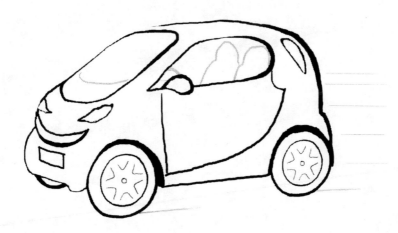

Colin …

By now most people see the picture: Climbing the mountain with a life partner with whom they maintain a mutually respectful, inspiring, motivating and encouraging relationship is preferred to being in a disharmonious, conflict ridden, or even hostile relationship.

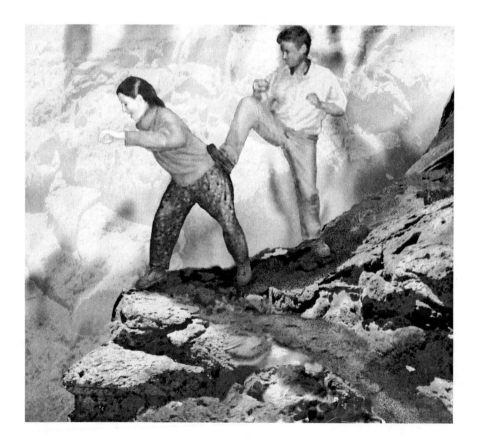

Ariole ...

So you - we - encourage people to take climbing courses?!?

Colin ...

I encourage people to create alliances with their partner, and to become conscious of the fact that being human includes being involved in a lifelong process of learning and moving forward.

Ariole ...

This is, perhaps, the centerpiece in a good relationship. Understanding - as a core awareness - that our partner is our greatest ally in our personal growth, learning, and development can be the most important discovery at the outset of a healthy relationship. This awareness can take place at the front end of a relationship, or it can be gained - like a 'dawning', a new light of consciousness - midway through the relationship. Either way, it will transform the very being of the two people involved. Not to mention the powerful 'ripple effect' that this new awareness creates around them through their new feelings, thoughts, speech, and behaviour. They begin to radiate and emanate joy, trustworthiness and leadership, showing others how and what a relationship can be.

Colin ...

Ariole, what do you think most people want in a relationship?

Ariole ...

I feel - even more than I 'think' - that people want to be respected. They want to be accepted for who they are, as they are. And through this respect they yearn to unfold the radiant beauty which is inside of them. This beauty is already inside of everyone. Just like a seedling - a plant - it needs to be loved and nurtured in order to grow and become resplendently evident.

Colin ...

How do people grow?

Ariole ...

They grow by seeing in themselves - or someone else seeing in them - their capability, their full potential in any given instant or situation or opportunity. This 'seeing' holds the space for them to grow into their full potential - their radiant beauty. Sometimes holding the space by seeing someone else's potential requires us - it 'calls' us - to challenge them. To catalyze them into new action, new thoughts, and new feelings about themselves. Our greatest ally is sometimes the one who challenges us the most. The difference between a healthy and an unhealthy relationship is that in a healthy relationship the trust - and the consciousness - exists for partners to challenge each other in a context of great love.

Colin ...

That's how we climb the mountain together, isn't it? By supporting each other through our ups and downs. When things are difficult, instead of pushing our partner over the edge, we can look up, smile, and say something like ... "I know it's a challenge. It's not easy. But let's get on with it. We're meant to succeed."

Becoming Allies
- Honest and Respectful
Communication

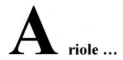 riole …

It's really important to understand the distinction between helping, supporting, and challenging your partner (or your friend, or anyone for that matter) in a healthy, ally way versus doing this in a codependent way.

In codependency we are agreeing - often without even being aware of this or discussing it outright - to keep each other as we are: small and 'safe'. With best intentions we keep each other in familiar territory *even if it isn't healthy for us.*

In a healthy relationship, we are each strong enough to challenge and be challenged. In fact, with every occurrence of challenge between partners, the relationship becomes stronger. And it is evident to both partners and to the honest people observing them that they are growing, that 'something is different about them', that they are becoming more courageous, more truthful, more direct, more in love.

Colin ...

In love with life.

People who suffer from bad relationships lack in some way in their love for life. They have withdrawn from hobbies and interactions with people. Their values, their inspirations, and their lives have become dull or rigid. The more we love life, the more we respect life. Love and life are the same. The more we love, the more we live. So the more we respect life, the more we respect love and thus treat our life partner with more reverence and dignity. This can be learned.

It can be learned by being honest. By making a conscious effort to be truthful. Because the moment that we're honest with our partner, we treat them with respect.

Ariole ...

And ourselves. We treat ourselves with respect. ... It's reciprocal. That's the nature of healing. What we extend to someone else is what we receive. There is no separation between we and they. What we give, we simultaneously receive.

That's the union. That's when we begin to truly create one energy field - a shared energy field - the 'union' which so many people aspire to. This is 'the peak' - the place where our two mountains join.

Colin ...

That's right. And isn't that what we all want? Oneness. And the moment that we're truthful, by being honest, we are in oneness. Because truth never has more than one side to it. So by being honest with your partner, you experience oneness with that person even when you disagree. Thereby, you can disagree without conflicts.

Ariole ...

I'd like to share an example from my - our - personal experience to illustrate Colin's point. In the first year or so of our relationship, there were a few times when I felt very strongly inside myself - a bodily sense - that I couldn't move forward with Colin without discussing something with him. Usually it was something he was doing or saying - or not doing or saying - which disturbed me. I was never quite sure whether it was 'his stuff, or mine'. Regardless, I knew that if I did not speak with him about this it would create an invisible wall of disharmony between us. And this would eat away at our trust.

I was always anxious about these discussions - the need for them, and the courage it required of me to address them.

What I discovered, to my amazement and sheer delight, was that Colin and I could truly listen to each other. Each of us had already done a lot of personal growth and self discovery. We were at a place of maturity - of ability to respect each other despite our differences - even when the other was showing us something about ourselves that we weren't aware of, or that they didn't like.

So first and foremost, we were able to truly listen to each other.

What happened, each and every time, was that we learned from each other in these conversations. Because we were always open and honest in our communication we grew enormously as a result of this process. We ended our conversations with a shared awareness of how to proceed - what each of us would do to create a better, mutually inspiring outcome. And ... we were closer, more in union, as a result of our clear commitment to peace and harmony.

After the first couple of these discussions I realized that there was nothing to fear in my disagreeing with Colin. I quickly came to trust that, if I ever felt uncomfortable about anything relating to him, I could speak with him about it. He would hear me. And I him. We became even more creative together. Through our inspiration and our commitment to grow, individually and as a couple, we became closer every day.

Colin ...

I agree. This is an example of being allies. What really works in our favor is our ability to communicate effectively with each other.

Ariole ...

To have the courage to speak, and the ability to hear. If we don't speak, there is no communication. So the communication begins with the person who is aware that something needs to be said, to be discussed.

Without communication - including exploration and expression of differences - walls grow. They accumulate. And they can become very difficult to penetrate and to untangle. It's far more effective for the health and joy of a relationship to learn how to communicate, rather than to default to the creation of walls.

It's about prevention, rather than fixing after the fact. Wounds can take a very, very long time to heal. Conscious couples know how to communicate rather than defaulting into the creation and augmentation of wounds.

Colin ...

Again, it's about being honest. We must deal with the fact - that something's wrong - when the fact arises. What I find is that a lot of people lack effective life skills. They mismanage their lives, and the resulting stress negatively affects their love life. Coming back to the principle of life balance, if a person lacks effective money management skills, their financial neglect will sooner or later negatively affect their relationship.

Whose marriage isn't affected by financial worries?

The question is, when did they not take financial action? Who was not honest about their financial affairs? Where and when did pride or greed get in the way?

Being honest with oneself is not easy, yet it is non-negotiable if one seeks a higher quality of life. Being able to face the fact and live the fact is an essential character quality if one aims to play the Game of Life at a higher level.

The Game of Life

C olin ...

I'd like to introduce another Coaching tool that I show my clients. It's called 'The Game of Life'.

Imagine you're participating in a game of tennis. You're on one side of the court, and life is on the other side. Life serves you a ball, and this ball lands in front of you, representing a fact of life. Such as ... you just got fired. Or promoted. What do you do about it?

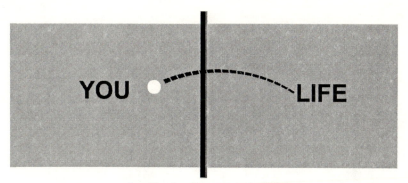

balls in front of you

What you do about the facts of your life - and what you don't do about the facts of your life - affects the quality of your life and your relationships. How many people do we know who have their courts cluttered with balls because they're not appropriately taking care of the facts of their lives?

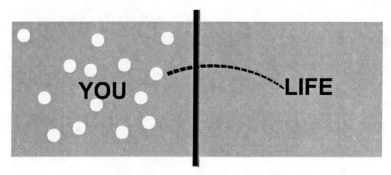

balls that you don't return

How many people do we know who look at the balls that have passed them, wondering what might have become of them?

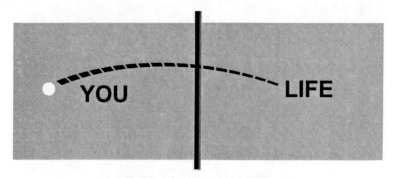

balls that may pass you by

How many people do we know who are missing the new balls that are landing right in front of them, right now?

How many people do we know who are staring across the net, worrying what balls might come their way?

Taking this idea back to relationship, how many people live in the past and don't see the beauty that's right in front of them in their life partner?

The solution-focused approach to one's life includes facing what's in front of me and dealing with it to the best of my ability. If my best isn't good enough, I hire a Coach and work on my 'inner game'. This includes the daily practice of Meditation.

Being Present - Meditation as a 'Way of Life'

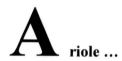 **A** riole ...

I teach Meditation - partly because altered states of consciousness and heightened awareness come naturally to me and partly because, in the day-to-day activity of my mind, I too need to learn how to be still. To bring peace to my mind.

In the practice of Meditation, it is quickly evident how little of the time a western human is actually in the present moment. I emphasize western, because in our culture we have come to over-value the thinking power of analysis and under-value the wisdom of the body, heart and spirit. To access these, we must know how to use our mind effectively and also how to still it. How to 'silence it' in order to 'hear', to sense, to feel, to know, to 'remember' the deep wisdom which our body / heart / spirit always have to offer us. They wait patiently for us to notice them.

Colin ...

Lack of stillness creates a real problem in relationship. 'She' worries about what might go wrong in life. 'He' fantasizes about sex. The practice of Meditation offers a simple solution to solve the root conflict of people's relationships. Too much thinking, too little loving.

Ariole …

Colin is a master at this - at recognizing when someone is thinking. He can see it in my eyes when I'm not present. He can feel it in my body. He instantly knows when I've 'left' the present moment. And thankfully for me, he is very gentle in bringing my attention to this - and thus calling me back into this moment, now. The only moment which is 'real' - the present.

Colin …

I have to thank Barry Long for teaching me how to be present, particularly being present in intimacy. He teaches lovers to be present with each other through eye contact. The moment that a person drifts away, you can see it in your lover's eyes. And if you're present enough to recognize this, you can gently request that he or she returns to the Now.

And that's where the tennis game that I referred to earlier becomes a great practice model for living in the now. Look at what's in front of you in terms of the facts of your life, and begin to deal with them. Now. By taking this approach to your life, you actively practice being in the Now. And you will thereby also learn to be present with your lover.

Ariole ...

This is such a powerful aspect of your wisdom and your teaching, Colin. Speak more about why worry in 'She' and fantasizing in 'He' are so detrimental to a relationship.

Colin ...

When she worries and he fantasizes, they are not together. Actually, they are both caught in their selfishness. They're both thinking about what they want and what they might not get. So both are attached to their desired outcomes. Neither one is giving to the other. They are caught up in the 'me' game. A good relationship is about 'us'. It's about him. It's about her. And also it's about me.

So when she worries - about what might go wrong with the children or the grandchildren - she is caught up in her own fear of possibly suffering and of not getting life satisfaction. When he fantasizes about sex, he's caught up in his own game of self-gratification.

Ariole …

Both are suffering.

Let's speak about how a woman can stop worrying. How a man can stop fantasizing.

Colin …

People can do many things, such as … take a Meditation course. Start a new hobby. Get involved in volunteering. Do something that keeps them in the moment.

Ariole …

Intriguingly, rock climbing is great for this - keeping the mind in the moment. So is white water kayaking. Ping pong. Any activity that requires millisecond to millisecond awareness of 'what is in front of you'. Anything that naturally 'yokes' the body / mind, uniting them for the purpose of quick and clear response.

Colin …

If you worry, start taking care of your cluttered life. If you fantasize, stop looking at others as a pleasure source. It is totally inappropriate for men to look at any female as a source of pleasure unless they have a relationship which includes expressed consent on her part.

Ariole ...

Yes, rape can be psychic just as it can be physical. The fear - fear of 'men' - which is held so deeply in the female psyche is very much a result of this. Boundaries, and their violation, exist on the etheric and on the physical levels. To respect other human beings is to respect them in their entirety - not just what you see before you - rather, all of who they are.

Colin ...

Women must also contribute to the solution. Women ... stop selling yourself in order to receive security in return. Stop playing into the fantasy world of men. Stop hooking men with promises you won't keep.

Ariole ...

Like a cat playing with a mouse, taunting it.

I once did an energy healing session with a man, and one of the most predominant 'alarm lights' resonating from his body was around the area of his penis. I discussed this with him. He said that he had had numerous sexual experiences in which he felt like he was held hostage by the woman.

Respect goes very deep. True respect knows no limits - it is infinite.

Women must respect men in order for their relationship with 'Man' to heal. And men, in the depth of their collective psyches, must heal to ultimately respect 'Woman'. For it is this respect which makes us ultimately trustworthy to each other. The terror and protection / defense against rape which exists in the collective unconscious of all women is twofold. Both women and men are responsible for cleaning up the lines of respect between both genders.

I am speaking here of all men and all women. Boys who will become men, and girls who will become women, too. That which is in our collective gender psyches permeates us all, often without us having any awareness of it. Peace - between man and woman - is the responsibility, and the ultimate creation, of us all.

Colin ...

Absolutely. Man and woman have co-created the world as it is today. And instead of complaining and blaming, the solution to our problems requires that we take responsibility equally for playing our part.

How can we do this? Again, take care of the unfinished business that's in front of you. Clean up your life. Because your life is your responsibility. Watch your temptation to blame and complain about how hard you have it. Just watch it. Don't be it. Don't become the complainer. Don't become the blamer. Don't be the victim.

Ariole ...

'Watching' is the Observer Mind, something we discover and fortify through Meditation. It is our ability to observe without reacting. When we observe, we shed light on what was previously unconscious. As the Buddhists point out, everything is impermanent. And so as we observe, we notice that things shift, they change, they dissolve, they resolve. Like nature - it's in constantly changing cycles. This is *natural*. When we react, we entrench things. We freeze them. In our culture, this has become 'normal'.

Colin ...

Yes.

Another thing you can do: Seek the ally who is seeking you. And begin climbing the mountain together.

If you are in a relationship now, speak to your partner about this. Ask your partner to become your ally. If you are single, look for someone with whom you can reach the top of life.

Ariole ...

Colin, you'd mentioned to me earlier that you'd like to define what a 'failed' relationship is - and isn't.

Colin ...

Sure. Failure is not necessarily failure. How is a marriage breakdown more of a failure than remaining in a dysfunctional relationship?

So what, then, is failure?

Failure is not doing the right thing. Failure is the fear - being frozen in the fear which keeps us from acting appropriately, honestly, compassionately.

Ariole ...

So as long as you're staying true to yourself, and to the 'tennis balls of life in front of you', you're not failing. You're very likely growing, which may seem like 'failure' because you're *changing*. Change may be labeled failure by others who don't like it. If you're true to yourself, and to the growth which life is calling you to play, then you're actually succeeding ... even if it doesn't appear that way to the worldly, judgmental bystander. All they see is people failing, and winning ... the state of duality. Love and mature, healthy relationships are beyond duality. Union is beyond duality. When a couple begins to live and grow together as a respectful union there is change and evolution, yet never failure or winning.

Colin ...

That's right. It's not about winning. What is winning anyway? Our society is so indoctrinated with the belief that someone must win. Unfortunately that requires someone else to lose. When people take this attitude into their relationships it sets up a system wherein nobody wins, and everybody loses. In real love, there is no winning or losing. People either spiral up or down. That is all.

Ariole ...

In fact, when people take the principle of winning into their relationship, they are automatically creating their partner as their adversary. The game - the relationship - is against them. As long as the egos - rather than the souls - are leading the relationship, there is a struggle for power, for 'rightness'. This can never succeed. It can only bring misery.

The Soul and The Ego

Colin ...

How can a person tell whether it is their soul or their ego which is leading the relationship?

Ariole ...

When you are able to act selflessly, it is your soul leading you. When you act for your own best interest (or perceived best interest), even if it depletes you or your partner, you are leading from your ego. Your ego is your identity of yourself as a limited human, as a person limited to your beliefs and ideas. Your soul is infinite and leads you by its very nature beyond the limitations of your ego. It is always leading you to grow, to become more of who you truly are.

If a relationship brings out the best in you, it is a 'soul' relationship. If it diminishes you or holds you in bondage as who you are now - who you 'appear' to be - then it is an ego relationship.

True union is always the union of two souls.

A simple 'radar' for choosing a soul partner is to seek someone whose nature it is to encourage you, to believe in you, to trust you, and to champion you to your greatness. They will help you to burst through your limitations, in a soul-full way.

Colin ...

This reminds me of Gary Zukav's definition of a spiritual relationship which he describes in his best-selling book <u>The Seat of the Soul</u>. A spiritual relationship is one that has the potential to serve as a framework enabling two people to reach the top of the Mountain of Life.

This really is about consciousness. The Mountain of Life is synonymous with ascending to higher levels of consciousness.

Climbing a mountain together requires self-knowledge, courage, willingness, forgiveness, acceptance, understanding and most of all - and this really is the most crucial element of it all - reverence for life. Feeling at awe ... when we contemplate ... the beauty of the mountain ...

Why would one want to ascend the mountain? If you've ever been hiking, you may remember that the higher you climb, the more pristine it gets. You meet familiar folk. The higher you climb, the smaller are the chances that someone's going to steal your food or wrestle with you.

The farther you go up, the greater are the possibilities that someone will stop and help you in a situation of crisis, or encourage you to reach higher heights when your fears seem to paralyze you.

The higher we climb, the more we experience union, togetherness, friendships, alliances, and unconditional support.

Ariole ...

That reminds me of real-life climbing again! It's not just a metaphor! When people rock climb, or climb mountain peaks, they are so encouraging of each other. Fear sets in, yes, often in the ascender. Inner fears surface which must be 'burnt off', evaporated by the ascent itself. And other people also climbing recognize this. Anyone who knows the territory of fear - of the 'unknown' - respects this in others. This respect is deep. It is a recognition both of the nature of fear, and of the tremendous freedom gained by piercing through it.

When we climb higher, we find our kin. We meet those who 'know' us - and have the potential to know us - in our core, the most precious place within us. We are no longer superficial strangers. We are soul friends.

Colin ...

At this stage of the 'game' you know you can't do it alone and you become aware that we're all equals.

It really helps to take your partner off the pedestal that you once placed him or her on, and realize that he or she - like you - is engaged in a lifelong process of climbing and learning and is thereby entitled to make mistakes - just like you are.

Ariole ...

Two things come to mind here. The first is that in most relationships people unconsciously, unknowingly, project their 'prince' or their 'princess' on their newfound date - or mate. They project onto - just like putting a mental 'costume' on a doll - their perception of who their ideal mate would be. When the person in front of them begins to show their humanness, their wounds and weaknesses - their 'flaws' - it becomes clear that they have 'failed' the projection. They are not the imagined 'prince' or 'princess'. They are a frog or froggess with warts.

This is where lovers turn to haters who resort to selfish blaming and complaining. And when relationships end with bitter feelings, the drama usually continues. A person may close their heart in cynicism towards potential future relationships or carry forward shields and armor - 'the past' - into the next episode of their own soap opera.

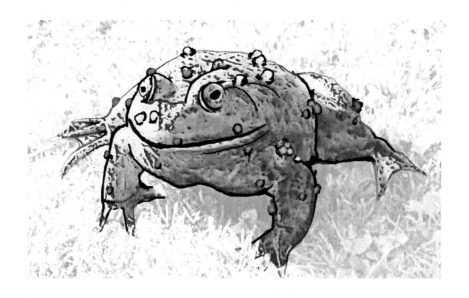

Colin...

You articulate this so clearly. Say more.

Ariole ...

This is the saga of most relationships now. They are not now. They are not real. They are not present. They are the imagination deceiving the mind. They are the mind creating misery, over and over again.

This is the 'Wheel' - the un-balanced one.

To awaken to this is to get off.

Getting off can look like this: Becoming your partner's ally.

When Colin and I met he was already well versed in Dan Millman's <u>The Life You Were Born To Live</u>. In it Dan brilliantly outlines, based on a person's birthdate - their 'birth path' - what their greatest life challenges, obstacles and opportunities are.

What happens in most relationships is that people instinctively know each other's weak points. Yet, because weak points signal that a person is not 'perfect' - not 'the princess or the prince' - *they attack them.* In the very places where your partner needs your greatest support and understanding, you are most likely to attack them.

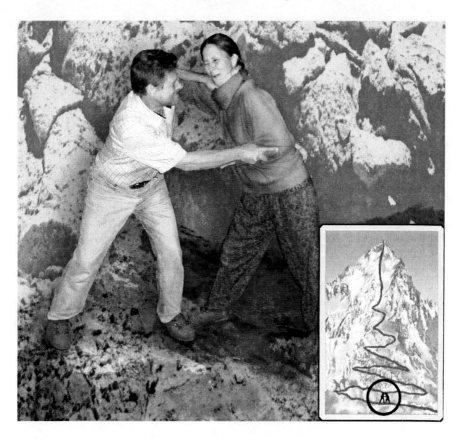

Until you become conscious. Until you become mature enough - and eager enough - to recognize your own and your partner's greatest life challenges. With this awareness you gain sensitivity and compassion. You realize that when your partner is facing the most difficult situations, behaviours and thought patterns, these are precisely the moments when you, as their trusted ally, can help them most to grow.

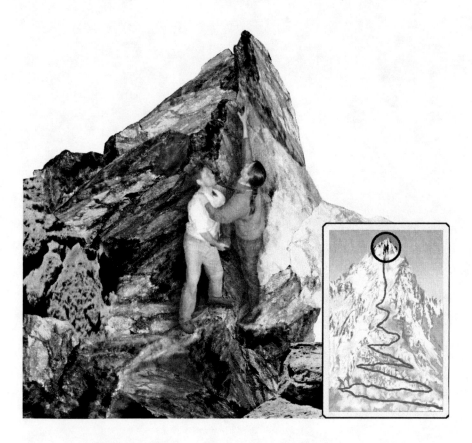

In recognizing their challenges you hold the space for them to learn from these and transcend them. You discipline yourself (if necessary) from ridiculing them - or gossiping about them to your friends. Instead you have compassion for them. Not pity. Compassion. You know - 'with' them - that they can ascend above this challenge. Together you find the solution, the creative answer, the new perception - the 'cure'.

Recognizing, with the assistance of <u>The Life You Were Born To Live</u>, what Colin's and my greatest life challenges are set a new frame of reference for our relationship right from the beginning. I was able to recognize how Colin played his challenges out. And rather than putting him down, belittling him, criticizing him, I was able to honor and respect him.

In the seven years that we have been together he has grown so incredibly. And so have I.

The fascinating thing about life challenges is that they are also the 'doors behind which our greatest gems lie'. In transcending them we unlock tremendous authentic power, confidence and clarity. We become more awakened humans.

Breaking the Chain of Abuse

C_{olin ...}

Often I encounter with my clients women who have been in a series of abusive relationships. A key issue for these women is how to deal with their past in order to have better relationships in the present. What I've found through the Coaching process is that we don't necessarily need to revisit the past in order to have a better future from now on.

Ariole ...

Yes. With powerful Coaching modalities we no longer need to 'heal the healing'. We can assist people to move directly into the future from an empowered present which is discovered and experienced through the Coaching process. I might add that it is an absolute joy and privilege to witness people move effortlessly into new futures without years of therapy and struggle. We always look for Coaching and Healing modalities which are effective on a source - rather than a surface - level and which are gentle, non-intrusive, and respectful. We've found and developed a number of these. It's a gift to work with them.

Colin ...

I completely agree. Here's an example.

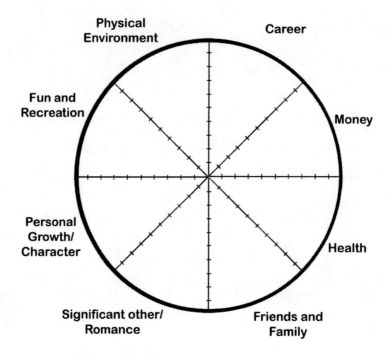

The 'Wheel of Life'

I recently had a sixty-two year old female client whose overall life balance was excellent. In our first session we reviewed her Wheel of Life and her scores in each of the areas were between eight and ten. She happily spoke about how good her life is as we were reviewing her Wheel - until we came to the area of relationship. She immediately admitted that this was her trouble spot. My sense was that this would be a deep session.

What she revealed was that she had been in a twenty-seven year long abusive marriage that included physical, emotional, and sexual violence. As we went on with the session she began to talk about the abuse that she had suffered in her childhood, including sexual molestation from her father and brother and rape at the age of sixteen. Her despair at this point was her uncertainty as to how to break the chain of abuse in her life. We began speaking about the two relationships she had been in since her marriage which also involved abusive men, though to a lesser degree.

The point I'm trying to make here is that in our first Coaching session we immediately explored how to put an end to receiving abuse, now. And what we found was that a person does not have to fight or be angry or be aggressive in order to stop abuse coming their way. All a person has to do is to be clear to stay away from conflict situations.

Ariole …

That's an assertive, non-aggressive way of setting a boundary. It is a declaration made by a person's inner Sovereign, articulated by their Magician, asserted by their Warrior, and given life - the meaning of life - by their Lover.

Colin ...

Yes. The inner Archetypes are a great way to explore and comprehend this.

Let me explain further. While this client's current partner was respecting her sexually he had been abusing her on occasion verbally. Her response at times was to strike back. So when we explored what it would be like to be in a relationship with someone who was not striking towards her, it became clear to her that she would then no longer be in a zone of aggression and there would be no reason for her to be aggressive herself.

I use a whiteboard in my office for illustrative purposes.

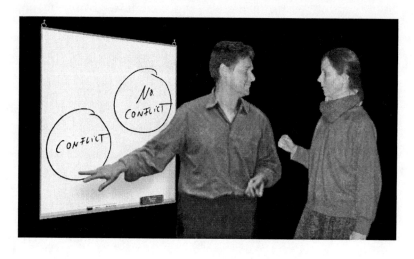

Colin …

I drew two circles. One said 'conflict' and the other 'no conflict'. Then I asked her, "Which of these two zones would you prefer to be in?" Her immediate response was, "The no conflict zone."

She began then to see that a powerful step for her would be to stay clear of conflict zones and conflict situations with people. To select relationships with people who do not seek, produce, or create conflicts.

She also spoke about how in conflict situations she would immediately clamp down, and that it would take her hours or days to open up again. We spoke about how difficult it is for women in society to deal with the bullying of men and that the natural response of a woman is to hide in her shell in order to avoid further strikes, blows, pain and suffering.

When she began to understand that her shutting down was a natural response to the threat from her environment and - taking this a step further by adding the fresh realization that she could choose her own environment - she felt a new sense of empowerment. She understood that by consciously staying away from conflict situations she no longer needs to shut down and hide. She also began to realize that in order to experience this improvement in her quality of life she no longer held a need to receive an apology from her ex-husband which, at the beginning of this session, she said she so much wanted.

Another important point to mention here is the common difficulty which women who are self-proclaimed Christians have in their relationships. They always feel inferior to men. This client said she tolerated the abuse from her partners because, according to the Bible, it is wrong to be angry with a friend. While it is not my role to change people's belief systems it is my responsibility as a Coach to help them have more clarity. And the clarity in this situation was about differentiating between anger and assertiveness.

What she and I agreed upon pretty quickly was that there is no excuse for disrespectful behavior by a man towards a woman. And that one does not have to become angry to stop inappropriate behavior. Rather one must, out of self respect, assert clear boundaries which require one to take a stand - towards integrity.

So in order to stop abusive behavior, a person does not have to lower themselves to the abusive, disrespectful nature of their aggressor. They must instead begin from an inner conviction that their aggressor's behavior is intolerable, inexcusable, unwanted, and no longer acceptable.

What changed for my client in this situation was that when she made an inner declaration that abusive, violent behavior was no longer an option for her in her relationship, she became clear not to compromise on her relationship any more. And this was a significant step for her in the process of completing her past and living more in the moment in a way that she had longed for ever since she could remember.

What I just revealed to you all took place within about sixty minutes.

The point I'm trying to make is that we can resolve the traumas of the past by doing what is right in the present moment, by choosing integrity.

The biggest point in this whole Coaching / Healing conversation with this particular client was really this: No woman should ever settle for anything less than respectful attention from any man.

It is no surprise that Dan Brown's The Da Vinci Code is an international, virtually instant bestseller. The Code's message that the sacred union between Man and Woman holds the key to heaven inspires millions of people around the world. It resonates with our personal yearning for truth and in so doing, it unlocks higher states of consciousness within us.

New Paradigm Relationships

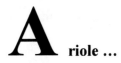 riole ...

I had an intuitive awareness when I was a young girl that ... it was better for me to not be in relationship than to be in a relationship that would keep me small. I immediately realized that relationships are meant to grow us. That when, in my future, I met a man whom I was attracted to I would only enter into a relationship with him if I felt that I could become *more* of myself. If not, I would not enter it.

I also saw an image of a healthy relationship as being like two trees. Each person is a tree. The trees are close enough together that the branches intertwine, yet far enough apart that they are their own people, with their own life experiences. The beauty of a healthy relationship is that we augment each other with our experiences, our insights, and even our opinions and beliefs. We stretch each other outside of our former shells. We bring out the best in each other - revealing the diamond hidden within.

For in the intimacy of a relationship built on respect and trust, it is our partner often who sees who and what we are capable of. We may have glimmers of this. Yet there are parts of us that are invested in us not changing. Sometimes we have the clarity and inner power to overcome the will of these parts. Sometimes it is the 'vision' of our partner which burns through them, as if opening the door of a hidden cage.

When I met Colin, I knew intuitively that I could complete my healing with him. That I could become my Self.

Colin …

Unlike you who was aware of the growing potential of relationships from an early age, I did not realize that relationships were meant for growth until I read Gary Zukav's <u>The Seat of the Soul</u> around 1994/95. Zukav's description of a spiritual relationship where two people unite for the express purpose of mutual growth created a contrast to the old paradigm of relationship that had as its primary purpose the insurance of mutual survival. In looking back I saw that virtually all disharmonious relationships and marriages that I knew of were still based in the survival model.

Ariole …

The childhood realization I described above led me to be single - with the exception of several short yet impactful learning relationships - until I was in my early thirties. I loved being single. I knew I was responsible for my own survival. And so I recognized the distinction between wanting and needing to be in relationship.

Spiritual Soul Parenting

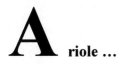 **A** **riole ...**

I also recognized as a child that most of the women in my culture were unconsciously programmed to believe that having children was a must. The drive to marry and have children was not even questioned by most. It was a 'given'.

I felt no need, recognizing this even as a child, to become a mother. In fact, I had a 'vision' in which I saw myself giving attention to thousands of people. I recognized the meaning of this vision to be that I (very probably) would not give birth to children. Rather, I would nurture thousands.

So this recognition that I didn't 'need' to either marry or become a mother set me free - enormously - to follow my own life path.

Colin ...

What is your life path?

Ariole ...

It is to awaken, and to encourage and assist others to awaken by touching their lives - directly and in the ripple effect - by my awakening.

I'd also like to say something about children. I've noticed from my view - we all have our own 'vantage' or angle from which we view every situation - that there are so many children born on this planet who are not truly loved. So few children it appears are truly, truly wanted. By this I mean wanted in a selfless way. So many children it seems are born to fulfill some wishes of the parents. So few parents love their children selflessly, with a conscious awareness of being stewards rather than owners of their children's lives. And then there are, too, the many, many children who are truly unwanted.

And so I believe it is vital that we begin to grow a cultural, human ethic that says it is a privilege to give birth or to father a child. It is a privilege, an honor, and a responsibility. It is perhaps the most important decision one can ever make.[1]

---

[1] See <u>Child Honoring</u> edited by Raffi Cavoukian and Sharna Olfman, 2006, www.raffinews.com.

Colin ...

Stewarding versus exploiting our children.

Ariole ...

I mean that we are the stewards of their souls. It is our responsibility as parents, extended family and friends, and the human culture as a whole to welcome spirits into this incarnate world and to guide them into the ways of the physical existence. This is a very sensitive process, one which - for virtually all of us - requires significant mentoring.

Colin ...

So true. We talked earlier about the Mountain of Life. If you are a parent reading these words, please reflect upon this idea ... Everybody was born to climb the Mountain of Life. There is only one Mountain of Life, yet it has infinite paths leading up to its peak. Within this context, everyone was born with a certain path - their life path - which leads them to the top of the Mountain of Life. If as a parent you can realize that your role is to assist your child(ren) to become strong 'mountain climbers', you are helping them to stay on their invisible path by gaining the life skills to successfully deal with the challenges and obstacles that are disguised as life learning.

Together, look for the clues - or open up the gates, and cross the bridges - which connect them to the next section or stretch of their individual life path.

Ariole ...

Colin, have you always had a concept of stewarding in relation to your children?

Colin ...

No. I have three boys from my first marriage. I've learned this concept through my own growth process which began around 1987 when I had none of the awareness that I am talking about in this book.

In 1987 I was struggling with ill health. In order to address some chronic conditions I decided not to go the medical route with drugs, but rather to pursue the natural way. When almost by coincidence a book on natural hygiene called <u>Fit for Life</u> fell into my hands ... At the university bookstore where I was returning a book on accounting theory! This marked a major turning point in my life because at this point in time I was wearing suits and ties and working as an accountant. I'd just started a new job and was sent away on a three week out-of-town training. This was fortunate for me, for in these three weeks I could provide my own meals and I had the opportunity to eat in the new way as described in Fit for Life. Within three weeks I lost twenty or thirty pounds and I felt and looked a lot better.

I was hooked. I began to read book after book on the subject of nutritional medicine and three years later I became a Certified Nutritionist and Iridologist. In 1990 I started to practice part-time and I transitioned into full-time holistic work in 1994.

My parenting style didn't change much until about 1995 when I discovered Dan Millman's system of lifepath numerology in his book The Life You Were Born To Live. Through his teaching I began to understand how we are all born with certain strengths and weaknesses, and I began to see my self and my children and other people through different eyes. Actually, I'd like to say I began to see people through a different heart.

This new awareness opened up my compassion for my children's 'misbehaviors'. And instead of addressing such misbehaviors by reprimanding them, I now focused on speaking to their potentials and strengths.

Dan Millman's work helped me to understand that on some level my children and I were in the same boat. We were equals. What differentiated us was only age, experience, and individual strengths and weaknesses.

I'm now convinced that our true role as parents is to provide an environment for nurturance through unconditional love and true justice.

Ariole ...

Yes. As we recognize that our parents and our children are souls - spirits - on the same shared infinite path of life as we are, the hierarchy dissolves. Who's to say who the older soul is? Or the wiser soul? So many of us have experiences of teaching our elders - not just practical things. I'm referring here to life lessons, principles of how the universe works, how energy flows, why we're here, what we've come for. Learning on that level of the 'soul'.

This is what makes relationships so deep, magical, and mysterious.

So true justice takes into account this broader perspective of who we are in relation to each other. People are not exempt from responsibility simply because they are older. Respect and trustworthiness are earned and maintained, moment to moment. They are based upon true character and consistent action.

Colin ...

How do we know as parents what's best for our children? How can we really know? If we don't even know what's best for ourselves? To be a good parent includes the humility to admit that one just doesn't know. What we do know, however - and this is evident moment by moment - is what is inappropriate. And then by addressing that, with wisdom and clarity and integrity, lies the application of unconditional love and true justice.

These principles are equally applicable to all spiritual relationships.

Ariole ...

There's something very interesting here. As we embark on the great odyssey of discovering what's best for ourselves - which requires that we come to Know our Selves - we naturally and reciprocally take our hands off the wheel of control of other people's lives. Because in gaining greater Self Knowledge we become humble, respecting the grace and uniqueness of everyone around us.

This may sound like utopia. The process of a human being awakening to their Self is an articulate process. The word 'process' is key. Just like a river with a strong current, wherein the forward motion of the surface is evident yet the back swirling undercurrents are unseen, our process of self awareness is similar. As more of the water becomes forward moving the natural arisal[2] of our humility as a consistent state takes place.

It is this humility that leads us into a recognition of parenting as a stewardship relationship rather than as ownership. This responsible guidance - with our controlling hands off the wheel of our children's (and our step children's) lives - is what spiritual soul parenting is all about.

---

[2] Often I find that words don't yet exist to accurately describe what is. And so I 'invent' them. Arisal is such a word. And so **arisal** *n* a birth, a rising upward of something new, an awakening into our perception or experience.

Unconditional Love and True Justice

C olin ...

Yes. And these same ideas are equally true for the man / woman relationship which is aimed towards attaining higher states of consciousness. We must learn to apply the principles of unconditional love and true justice in our love relationships in order to have the experience of complete satisfaction and fulfillment in our love lives.

The idea of spiritual soul parenting as we described it earlier is significant also to the way that we mentor ourselves through our everyday life. Because in many ways as adults we are our own parents. And the ignorance of this fact leads to our unaware, continued expression of the programming we received from our parents, teachers and mentors when we were children. The quality of this programming is equal to the level of consciousness of those people in the earlier part of our lives.

Weeding the Garden

C olin ...

Here it becomes very important to recognize what Ariole described earlier as the 'waking up'. Wake up to your programming. Look at how you habitually react to people and to life circumstances. Question your own belief systems. And above all, consider the possibility that your way of seeing it all might be wrong. Ask other people how they see you. If you have children, ask them, 'Please tell me what you see that's wrong with me.' And listen, from a neutral zone. Don't react to their answers. Rather ask yourself this question: 'What can I do about it?'

I call this process 'weeding the garden'. Or 'cultivating my energy field'. In Coaching a client will often say, 'Coach, I need your help to identify what I want.' When we begin this process of identifying what they want, often the common response is, 'Oh my God, this is so difficult. I'm so confused. There are so many choices. I don't know what I want.'

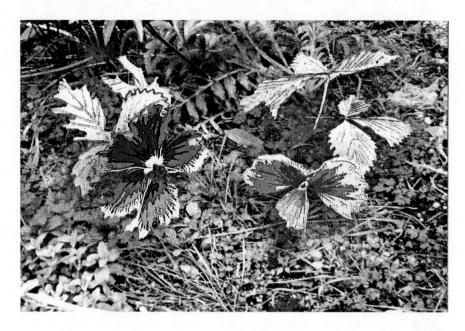

'Well, let's take a different approach', I say. Instead of identifying what you want, identify what you don't want. This is often much easier, because what you don't want you already have and thereby you have the power to do something about it. This is synonymous with facing the project of what to do with a wild garden. You may say, 'I don't know what to do. There are so many choices. Rose gardens. Fruit trees. Berry bushes. Japanese gardens. Potatoes.' You get the idea. The options are endless.

So why not start doing something about that which you don't want? Weeds. Begin by plucking the weeds. And lo and behold, as the weeds go, in comes the clarity of what you could do with that wonderful space.

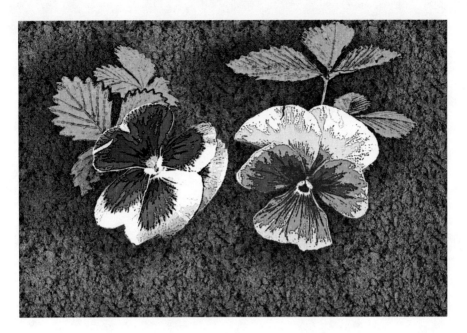

Colin ...

Now our life is not much different. Take your relationship for example. If your love relationship is not as good as you'd like it to be, instead of daydreaming of who you'd rather have in your life, address with your partner that which you don't want. And change it. Don't give up. Until the weeds are plucked.

This is one powerful way of creating a spiritual relationship. Because in the process of plucking the weeds, you are growing, and so is your partner.

Ariole ...

Because, just like in a real garden of 'plants', the fewer the weeds, the more light there is available - and soil, and space - for the chosen plants to grow. The chosen plants are the elements or qualities or dreams that you both willfully desire to nurture and to support.

Colin ...

Right on. And growing towards the light is the evolution of consciousness. To further that evolution of consciousness is the true purpose of a spiritual relationship.

Ariole ...

The 'garden' represents our shared life together, as a couple. It is what we are building, growing, fostering, nurturing - in being together, in sharing this life together.

Love and Respect
- the Antidote to Abuse

C olin ...

Earlier we talked about abusive relationships and what to do about them. We talked about how to make non-appropriate behavior a non-option in order to free ourselves from abusive relationships. But part of the problem - and this may be one of the reasons why people stay in abusive relationships - is that they don't know how to determine what is inappropriate behavior. For example, a person may dislike being yelled at or being reprimanded, but at the same time believes that he or she only deserves to be treated that way.

I recently had a client who had been in a string of abusive relationships including verbal abuse, and when she realized that she didn't need to be talked to that way anymore, it seemed easy for her to create a natural boundary because she now realized that what she didn't want she also didn't deserve.

The problem so often is that we continue to attract our parents' behavior from the days that we were little. There seems to be an ongoing, unconscious idea - like in this example: 'My parents told me and modeled to me that I need to be talked to in that way, and thereby I deem this to be necessary for the rest of my life, because this is who I am.' So early on in our life we create this personal identity and then continue to attract people into our life who treat us in exactly the 'right' way to affirm this self image.

Ariole ...

This stems from the fact that we raise children to follow the likes and wants of the parents. We don't really know, as a culture, how to raise children in a way that nurtures their recognition and understanding of who they are as sovereign entities, when they need boundaries, how to create them, and how to maintain them in a healthy way. How to be neither passive nor aggressive. Rather clear, confident, respectful of self and others, and assertive. Because we don't know how to do this, what we model to our children is a doctrine that the 'elders' are the rulers. This results in us learning, at a very early age and then consistently throughout our life, to give our power, our responsibility, and our decision-making to someone outside of us. How can we then know when we need boundaries, how to assert them, and how to manage them? We become, as Colin cited with his client, confused as to what is right and wrong. What are we entitled to and what do we 'deserve'?

So what is the solution? To teach our children differently. And ... because we are now 'adult children', we need to teach ourselves differently. We need to reclaim our power, our decision making, and thus our responsibility. Through this process we regain our clarity. We re-access our intuition and our instinct. Our intuition and instinct are our inborn ability to 'Know' what is right and what is wrong, what we must do and say and be in order to be truthful - to be in our integrity in every moment, in every situation. This is the process of being true to our Self, rather than to our conditioned self.[1]

Colin ...

The key to a fulfilling love relationship is love and respect. You'll end up in paradise if you 'weed your garden' well. Ask powerful questions: 'Is this respectful? Is this loving?' Coming back to the example given with the earlier client, when her partner yelled at her she could have asked herself, 'Is this respectful?' Her

---

[1] See the trilogy Awakening Instinct - the true feminine principle ♥ Running the Gauntlet – navigating our way to our fully embodied potential ♥ Windows Through Time - a 'possible evolution' story - also by Ariole K. Alei, HeartSong Solutions, 2006. Awakening Instinct is a 'treatise' which channeled through Ariole in one of her Meditation classes. Immediately afterword it asked her to 'transcribe' it as a book.

answer clearly would have been, 'No.' Most likely her inner judge would then have added, 'But you're a bad girl. You deserve to be corrected and punished.' Then she could have asked the question again, 'Yes, I understand. But is this respectful? Is this loving?'

You see, there is no excuse for being disrespectful and unloving. Yet in our culture we control people through what we call 'love'. Withholding love, yet still maintaining that one does love the person, is called conditional love - which is not love at all. It's pure bullshit. Nonsense. It's a lie!

Ariole ...

It's really manipulation. If we see it as what it is - not as what we're supposed to agree that it is - we recognize that it is self-serving manipulation.

Colin ...

Exactly.

Ariole ...

And this is what our culture is built on. This is the glue that holds it together. The sand beneath it. This is codependency. The invisible lies that present themselves as love.

Colin ...

The bottom line for a good relationship is love and respect. Love and respect must be non-negotiable. So if I ask the question, 'Is this respectful? Is this loving?', and the answer is, 'No', there is no justification required. Coming back to the earlier example with the client who had been in a string of abusive relationships, when she asked, as he was yelling at her, the question, 'Is his way of speaking to me respectful?' - and her clear answer was, 'No, it's not respectful', then - and this is very important to understand - the next right step is not to justify his behavior, but to create a boundary with it.

Ariole ...

This is the only way that we can create a healthy, truthful society.

Colin ...

Love and respect begin with one's self. It is important that we question our own behavior - towards our self and others - in this way. If there ever was any failure in a relationship - and I'm excluding now relationships which have stopped because they have outlived their usefulness - I like to suggest that the real reason for failure has been the violation of the principle of love and respect.

We could complete this book right here, if the reader were to fully grasp this principle of love and respect. That's how important it is. Why? Because love and respect are the foundation for a life of joy and peace. Isn't this what we all want? Joy and peace? We cannot have it without having love and respect first. This becomes obvious when we Coach clients along the 'Map of Consciousness' outlined by Dr. David Hawkins' in his milestone book <u>Power vs Force</u>. Transcending duality - suffering - requires reverence for life. This is unconditional love.

Ariole ...

It's simple to see this - to 'get' it - when we realize that love and respect are God, the creator, the Source, the All That Is. When we love and respect something, someone, ourselves, we are recognizing God in them and in us. When we recognize God in each other we can only be peace and joy. We can no longer be anything antithetical to this. War, hatred, jealousy, resentment - these states of thinking and feeling can no longer exist once we recognize ourselves and each other as God.

As with all deep, rich, core teaching, it is one thing to understand this conceptually. It is another to understand it in the whole of our being. When we 'embody' this understanding, we live it. And when we live it, our life becomes it - peace and joy.

Colin ...

That's right. There must be a practical application of what we have just said.

Let me give you, the reader, a practical demonstration of this right now. Please ask yourself this: 'Is the content of this book that I'm reading right now respectful of me and others? Is its message loving?' If you answer 'Yes' to either of these two questions, chances are that this book is useful to you. If your answers are 'No', I suggest that you immediately close this book and give it away. Because you should never, ever engage yourself with someone or something that is not loving and/or respectful. You should never, ever not be loving and respectful to yourself. If you want to improve the quality of your relationship(s) and have more joy and peace in your life, then love and respect are not negotiable.

Ariole ...

I teach my Meditation students and Coaching clients how to discern that which is loving and that which is not - how to differentiate them - by noticing what is life-affirming and what is life-negating. That which is life-affirming is inherently respectful and loving. That which is life-negating (draining, confusing, fatiguing, depleting) is not respectful or loving.

Once we recognize that something or someone - an event, a place, a food, an interaction, a source of information, an idea - is either life-giving or life-negating, we then know either to move toward it or away from it. In the latter case we sometimes, though not always, need to move away from it and create a boundary to it. This boundary is a clear 'No' which disallows it from engaging with us **until or unless it becomes loving and respectful to us.** Then we can dissolve the boundary and engage with it. For it has become, and now it is, life-giving.

Living in this way heals us, the human being, and our species. It is a very powerful thing. It's how we become true to ourselves - and to others. And this - this truth - is what respect is. Respect is being truthful. It is the absence of lying, of deception, to ourselves and to the world. It is being truth. Being truth. Truth.

Oneness
- Transcending the Human Shadow

C olin ...

This takes us into oneness. Because truth has no two sides. And oneness is what we all want, don't we? To end the painful sense of separation is to have oneness.

This is where an intimate relationship provides such an immediate response or feedback for the degree of oneness or separation that one has attained. A relationship that is based on mutual love and respect produces joy and peace, serenity and bliss. These states of consciousness ultimately lead to the highest level of consciousness - the realm of enlightenment. Enlightenment really is the state of shadowlessness, meaning there's only light and no shadow. Shadow is produced by disrespectful and unloving behavior, which we feel as shame and guilt, apathy and depression, fear and anger.

Ariole ...

Shadow is created when we try to hide something about ourselves - from ourselves and from others. We 'put it behind us', where we cannot see it, and where we hope to be able to deflect others' attention from it.

Shadow eats us. It eats our life force. Everything grows. And so we can understand that that which we cut off from our daily 'acceptable self' needs to be fed, too.

And so we live our lives feeding the visible and the hidden aspects of ourselves.

The simple way to end this - to resolve its 'side effects', of which there are many - is to be truthful. To be transparent. To tell only the truth - to ourselves and to the world around us.

When we live as if we have nothing to hide, something amazing happens. We become more than human - as we have come to believe humans are. We become, in fact, the true nature of Human. We become Light incarnate - benevolence, freedom, openness, radiance, infinite Love.

Colin …

The truth is, we have nothing to hide. If we think we can hide something, we live an illusion. You may be able to hide something from someone for a short period of time. But someone, sooner or later, will be awake - alert enough - to pierce through the veil.

Ariole …

The only reason we ever perceive a need to hide something 'about' us is because of a sense of guilt or shame.

Guilt plays a healthy function *when we listen to it and learn from it.* When we allow it to show us that we have done or thought or said something which is not respectful. When we accept this awareness and learn from it - thinking, saying, and behaving respectfully in the present and thus the future - we have no reason to feel guilty again. And so, with no reason to feel guilty, we feel no compulsion to hide ourselves.

Shame in the way that most of us experience it is unnecessary. Because we don't receive its message, we are crippled by it. Shame, if perceived and responded to *immediately,* is like a compass refining our course. It tells us when we have been incongruent, untruthful. Because most of us don't recognize this guiding power of shame, we wallow in it and allow it to drown us. Like water being pulled cyclone-like down a drain, shame sucks us into perpetual victimhood. It thus becomes a conditioned human response malevolently keeping us small. Shame keeps us from shining. It binds us into spending our precious life force in feeding our shadow.

There is nothing that *any* of us need be ashamed of. Shame which is not recognized as a 'beacon' and swiftly acted upon, like a captain of a ship, becomes a 'human' creation. A judgement. A crippling device.

When we bring forth from our shadow everything that we formerly hid *because we felt ashamed of it,* we begin to realize the fallacy of this. We begin to integrate all aspects of ourselves. We begin to realize that we are lovable - and that we always have been. Someone, sometime, may have reacted negatively to us. And we may have misinterpreted this and felt toxic shame.

Now is not the past.

As we bring into the light - into visibility, 'in front of us', what was our shadow, thus emptying it - we discover that people *do* love us. *Precisely for who we are.*

We are liberated from the unspoken expectation of our society that we will agree, without question, to carry a shadow.

How do you recognize a human? They have a shadow, a hidden darkness dragging behind them.

How do you recognize a Hu-man? They are completely transparent. And what's more, they *radiate Love.*

This is a practice. We must practice putting our shadow in front of us - and discovering that there is no need for shame, and thus no need for shadow. In doing this, we become Hu-mans, again.

Colin ...

When we feel shame, we feel humiliated, outcast, non-human, not worthy to be human, separate, the opposite of oneness. The immediate remedy to shame and humiliation is to return to love and respect and act with integrity. Healing our human condition of separation, of loneliness, can be as simple as that. Again I suggest to practice it right now. Every moment of your life is right now. Keep practicing asking the question, 'Is this respectful? Is this loving?' When you do this, you let love lead the way. And as you're following the way - the path – you're one with love. When you're one with love, you already have love. And it cannot be taken from you. Now you are free from the codependent nature of so-called loving relationships - which are really not loving relationships at all.[1]

---

[1] See also <u>The Mastery of Love</u> by Don Miguel Ruiz.

Loving from the Inside Out - Beginning the End of Human Suffering

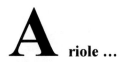 riole ...

Codependent relationships include covert, unconscious contracts - agreements - of suffering. They are master-slave relationships in which we are bound together to not disagree, allowing one person to believe they are in charge, dominant to the other, when in fact both people are slaves to the codependency.

This is so subtle that we, as a society, a human culture, do not recognize the scope and scale - the tangled web - of codependency that we have become as a species. In recognizing and practicing truthfulness - respect and love - we are untangling this sickly web.

Colin ...

In the master / slave relationship, no one wins. Even the master is a slave to the master / slave relationship. Because without the slave, he could not be a master. He therefore lacks his freedom to be who he really is. The master / slave relationship is devoid of love and respect. It thereby enslaves the master to the reality of separateness, because only love and respect enables us to transcend separation. And with separation we suffer.

Ariole ...

I heard myself asking a group of Meditation students a year ago ... 'When did you sign a contract to suffer?' We were all silent for some time, shocked by the simple poignancy of that question. When had we? We lived our lives as if we had! When had we? Pondering this question - piercing through the invisible 'rules' which bind us to limitation and separateness - is a primal, core, transformational experience.

When did you sign a contract to suffer?

Colin ...

We never did. But it seems that we were conditioned by our parents, mentors, teachers to live that way. So suffering is one way to live. But it is not the only way. There are other options. Let's just contemplate for a moment that suffering is one of the many options by which we can live and experience life.

So what are some of the other options? Non suffering? Non sacrifice? Truthfulness? Honesty? Respectfulness? Loving? Caring? Stillness? Why not choose one of these for a while. Just to test it. To do a little experiment. To see what happens when I wake up in the morning and I say to myself, 'Suffering is not an option.' So what happens when, later in the day, I trip and sprain my ankle, and I feel pain? Maybe even excruciating pain. Do I need to suffer? Of course not! Because the only time I suffer is when I get into the victimhood that says, 'You idiot! How could you have tripped?!' Or the poor me who says, 'Here I go again. Life's against me. It's all so bad. It's hopeless.' I'm now afraid that life will never be good for me, that I will never experience love, joy and peace. Instead of seeing that all that happened is that my body got hurt and now it is suffering.

But I'm not suffering. My body is.

What do I mean by this?

We're getting into a really vital conversation now of separating ourselves appropriately from the inside out. People so often make the mistake of identifying themselves with their body, their mind, and their emotions. An important point here is to acknowledge that, yes, there are painful conditions or situations, and they do hurt. But one does not have to suffer.

Ariole ...

I had a colleague once who experienced frequent stressful interactions with others. She asked me if I could see what the 'dynamic' was that repeatedly tripped her up. I couldn't see it initially, yet I promised to reflect on this and to share with her any insights which came to me. It was several months later - I was in India and she was miles away in England. I was shown this ... She was the catalyst for me to recognize a universal principle at play in humans.

When we are wounded, internally, in terms of emotional, psychological wounding, a part of us which is very young is deeply confused. The wound suggests that we are bad, dirty, unworthy. And yet the soul, which is present in each of us, continually knows and affirms that we are inherently good and love-able.

So the wounded part of us seeks situations to affirm its belief. In fact, it finds people and situations it can manipulate into the 'oppressor' role *so that its victim identity can be reaffirmed,* over and over again.

Thus people and circumstances are often manipulated *by us* to oppress us. Unless we are very awake to this and have very clear boundaries to this, thus disallowing ourselves to be manipulated in this way, we find ourselves in the equally confusing situation of appearing to be an oppressor, when this was not our intention or our interest at all.

Colin ...

This is so true. It is one of the hidden dynamics operating between so many people. It is at the root of codependent relationships.

Ariole ...

Suffering is falling into drama. It is asking the world around us, non-verbally, to feed - to give attention to - that which is 'broken'. Rather than asking for food - attention, support - to heal it.

When we choose to suffer, or when we join someone else in their suffering, or when we ask someone to join us in our choice to suffer, we are lowering the consciousness of ourselves and those we engage with. We are choosing to perceive ourselves as smaller than we really are. We are turning away from our true selves.

Colin ...

Suffering is a state of duality. We only suffer because we wish that things were different than they are. Suffering arises in a sheer state of ignorance due to non-acceptance of the facts of life.

For example, I arrive at the airport late. I miss the plane. Now I suffer because I wish it was different. So I hang on to an ideal, meaning that, 'I could be on that plane.' But the ideal is not reality. Because I'm not on that plane. So there's a source of suffering. Non-acceptance of a fact, wishing things were different, being in duality. Duality being, 'there's a fact, and there's the ideal.' In this example, duality being 'there's my plane in the air, here are my feet on the ground.' That's duality. Two points of reference.

The solution to this dilemma in this situation ... Forget about the plane. Be where you are. And ask the following question, 'What is the most important next step that the respectful, loving me could take?' The answer to this question will take you right into the action mode again and out of suffering. You have resumed the driver's seat of your life. You are in a co-creative mode, and you're happy. Your attention is in the now. And since there's only now, you're one with life. And when you're one with life, suffering is impossible, because life never suffers.

Ariole ...

Because life is God.

Colin ...

Yeah. Let's take all these ideas into the area of relationship.

If you're suffering in relationship, stop wishing it was different and do something about it.

Here's an idea of what you can do.

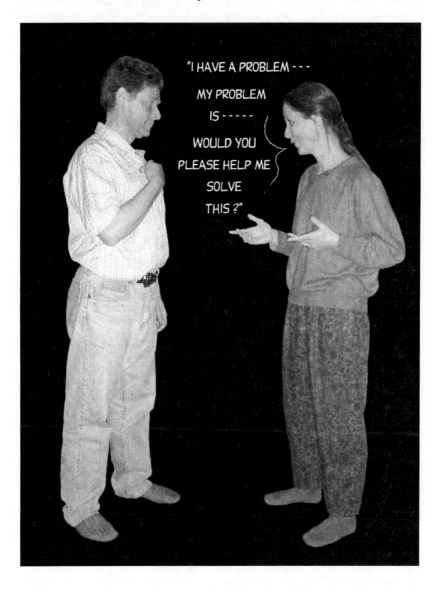

Make a list of the top ten problems in your relationship - from the way you see it, and from the way your partner sees it. If you're currently single, use the top ten problems from your last relationship and pretend they're in your life right now. Once you've written your list, ask yourself this question, 'What can I do about each of these problems? What are the top three steps I can take to solve each of these relationship problems?' As you ask these questions you will notice that some of these problems can be solved by yourself, and others can't. With problems that require the assistance of somebody else, identify who you need to ask for help, and then go to that person and say something like, 'I have a problem. And I'm asking you for your help to solve it.'

Then describe the problem and ask for the other person's input to solve it. Chances are the other person is a part of the problem. But by having identified the problem as your problem, you are no longer blaming or complaining to the other person. By taking ownership of the problem you are not in the victim role. You are in the process of empowering yourself and the other person to create a better life together by solving your problem as allies.

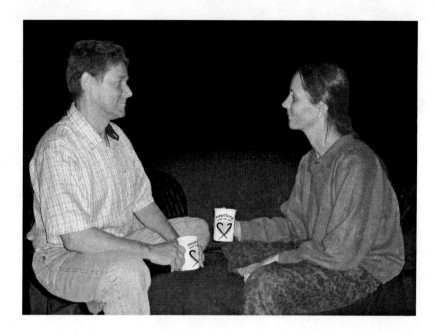

Communication
- the Enlightened Path

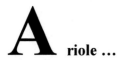 riole ...

It's been said often, and it's so true, that communication skills are at the core of a healthy, long and enduring, joyous relationship.

Colin and I are so fortunate to have discovered at the beginning of our relationship that we can speak with each other about anything. And, because we are mature enough to listen - and be humble to each other's wisdom - we always grow as a result of our 'challenging' conversations.

I realized years ago that if a relationship can withstand honesty, it is true and deep. If it cannot, then perhaps the honest conversation is the one that shows us, very clearly, that we have outgrown the relationship. This is true with friendships too. With any kind of relationship for that matter. If the relationship cannot allow us to be truthful - in a mature way, one which includes deep listening to the other person's point of view and experience - then it is not a relationship for us to carry forward with us.

This is another aspect of weeding the garden. Carrying forward with us only that which allows us to be truthful as we discover more and more the essence - the heart, the spirit - of who we truly are. Our relationships must continuously grow and become more authentic as we - a vital and active ingredient at the heart of these relationships - become more and more authentic, more and more true. If they do not, and we carry with us 'old' relationships - ones which we've outgrown - we allow them to deplete us. To prematurely age us. To keep us small. To support us in being dishonest.

If we are honest we are always growing, always waking up, always coming to know our Self more deeply. And with that strength - and recognition of our inner beauty - comes the willingness to let the old go.

Colin ...

Through being truthful we are maintaining soulful connections. And that's how we find our Soul Mate. The problem for so many people in relationships is that their actions and reactions, behaviors and feelings are governed by their rational mind. Out of fear. And not by their soul, out of love. And so people often remain stuck in relationships rather than moving forward and upward in the spiral of life towards more soul growth and healing. And as a result of being stuck they suffer the pain. Literally, from being stuck. Just like it would hurt if your foot or your finger was stuck somewhere. And the 'stuckness' would begin to cut off the blood supply, meaning the life force. This scenario is synonymous with what happens in relationships wherein people - out of fear - don't speak the truth because the truth would mean realizing the fact that now they need to experience the death of the relationship. And one of the greatest fears that humans have is the fear of death and dying.

Ariole ...

Even the way we hold our breath, being shallow breathers, high up in the chest, is an embodiment of our fear of death. We are afraid, as a culture, that life will not return to us with the new breath, with the next moment. And so we cling on to what we have (or perceive that we have) - including the old breath. That which was new and fresh in the moment and yet - as we hold on to it, when its natural course is to run through us and beyond us, 'out of us' - it becomes old, stale, dead.

And so we create death, by avoiding death.

This we do in relationships too. In our relationship with our self, to begin with. And then as a ripple effect, emanating out from this core dishonesty, in our relationships with life and with other people.

The natural course of all energy is constant movement. In nature, nothing is static. It may appear still, and yet it is not static. Because nature is not afraid of death. Nature allows energy to cycle as it will, creating, transforming, decaying, destroying and creating again.

When we learn to trust life, we allow death. Death is naturally occurring in and around us every moment. It is a natural phenomenon. To be truly alive, parts of us must be continually dying.

For a relationship to be truly alive, we must allow that which is no longer true, that which is no longer relevant, that which has become smaller than the new, current maturity ... to die. Only in allowing the small deaths can a relationship be fully alive.

This takes courage. And understanding. Yet it works. It always works. It is what keeps life real, what keeps life fresh.

Colin ...

Truth keeps life fresh.

Ariole ...

Exactly.

Colin ...

Truth is the one thing that frees us, liberates us, rejuvenates us and invigorates us. Yet it seems to be so hard to find. We alluded earlier to the importance of having effective communication skills and in my experience, one requires communication skills in order to find the truth. Many people in their relationships stop short of finding the truth of the matter because they just don't know how to look for it - how to find it. Because they don't know how to ask the right questions.

When two people have disagreements the most common outcome is conflict and frustration. Frustration is nothing but incomplete communication. Almost everyone wants peace, and peace we find when we have truth. So in order to find that truth when we are in a conflict situation, it helps to ask open-ended questions. Such as, 'What do you mean? Why do you say that? Who thinks that way? How can we solve this problem?' Instead of responding with defensive or aggressive statements.

Here's a simple diagram which is part of an effective communication toolkit. In Coaching language we call this communication system 'Logical Levels'. It is used to ask open-ended questions.

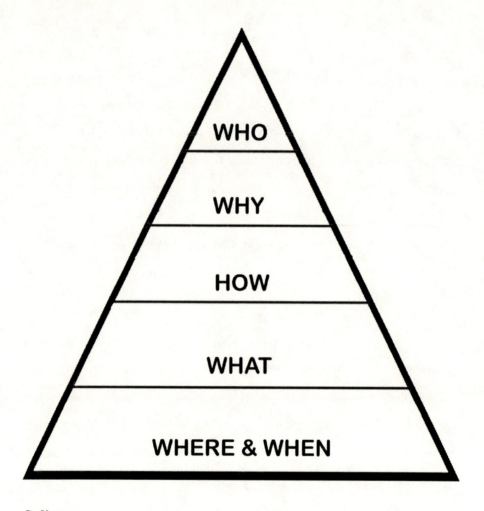

Colin ...

Here's an example of how one might use it. Your spouse comes home and accuses you of cheating. Your spouse is jealous, aggravated, and confrontational. Your standard response may be to be defensive and say something like, 'No I'm not.' Then he / she says, 'Yes you are!' And the debate heats up. Can you see where this leads?

Using the Logical Levels we can get a different outcome by getting to the truth of the matter. After your spouse's initial accusation or statement you could say, 'Why do you say that?' And then wait for the answer. Find out why your spouse really thinks that you are cheating. Is your spouse possibly projecting his or her infidelity onto you? Get to the truth of the matter. You could ask, 'How do know when someone cheats? What's the evidence?' Maybe you just smiled at somebody out of gratitude for their opening the door for you and your spouse misinterpreted this as flirting? Get to the truth of the matter instead of being defensive. Don't be afraid of what you might find. Dig to the point of oneness. Expose what's hidden. Truth is oneness. There's only one truth. That's when you have peace.

In our company **HeartSong Solutions**™ we place great emphasis on learning effective communication skills. I've taught many people the Logical Levels system with magnificent results.

Ariole ...

Truth starts with ourselves. If we are not truthful with ourselves, we cannot be consistently truthful with others.

Being truthful with ourselves requires, for many people, tremendous initial courage. For in turning 'inward' to see what has been hidden in our 'shadow', we have no conscious idea what we might find. Usually the fear is greater than the reality. And if we consider that everything in our shadow is a collection of the past, then we realize that - no matter what we may have done or said or not done in the past - this moment now is an opportunity to do and say and be different. If we are humble and willing enough to take responsibility for anything that we may have done in the past that was in any way harmful or negligent, then there is nothing to fear.

Everything in the past can be forgiven. Everything.

The first step in becoming able to be truthful in our relationships is becoming truthful with ourselves. If we are unhappy, then there is something that we are not being truthful about with ourselves. There is something that we are ignoring. When we listen deeply to the 'quiet, still voice within', we can know what is true for us. Maybe it is that we need to change careers, workplace, or home. Maybe it is that we have outgrown what was our dearest friendship. Maybe it is that our body has become sluggish and we need to make healthier food and exercise choices.

Maybe it is that we need to be more selective about the information that we allow into our very influential brain. Maybe it is that we said 'Yes' when our honest response would have been 'No'.

When we recognize that unhappiness - and illness - is a signal that we are being in some way dishonest with our self, then we can heed this signal, make a different choice, and become happy again.

When we learn to do this with our self - to have the courage to see what is real with us - then this becomes much, much easier to do with other people. It becomes no longer a matter of courage, rather a matter of simply doing it. Of being honest.

Barry Long calls this "being straight".

Colin ...

Barry Long also said, "I cannot teach you enlightenment. But I can teach you honesty." By being honest we are finding the truth and only the truth, and this enlightens us.

Being honest first requires us to become honest. And we become honest by practicing honesty. How do we practice honesty? By being more respectful. How do we become more respectful? By asking ourselves this question often, 'Is this respectful?' For example, you are in a relationship with someone and you are not stating the truth, maybe it is that you don't love that person anymore. But this person says to you, 'I love you.' And you say, 'I love you too.' Are you being respectful? You may respond, 'Well, I don't want to hurt that person's feelings.' But how do you know that you would? How do you know that telling a lie hurts less than telling the truth? Is the truth of the matter not that you're trying to avoid your own pain and suffering that may result from facing up to the truth? Which in this example is that you don't love this person anymore, you want to get out of the relationship, which requires the process of separation, which brings on change, and your perception is that this type of change always brings on pain and suffering. So you avoid being honest in order to avoid getting hurt. How selfish is that?

Recovering from the
Politics of Love
- Selfless, Soulful Loving

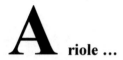 **riole ...**

We seem to hide so much selfishness in the general model of relationship in our culture. Either we're being codependent, which is selfish, or we're being outright selfish, which is selfish. The first is covert - hidden - the second is overt - visible. What is selflessness in the context of relationship? Let's talk about that. Let's paint a picture of how to be in a relationship without being selfish.

Colin ...

It's easy. Just be honest. Just be honest. By being honest, you surrender to an idea that's greater than the selfish 'you'. Integrity. Honesty. Truth.

The small selfish part will always try to deceive, to trick, to manipulate, for selfish gain. The noble self will always be honest and true, regardless of the short-term effects. Because it knows that long-term peace can only be attained by being honest.

Ariole ...

There's something about being congruent - about being honest on all four levels of our being. The physical, emotional, mental, and spiritual or causal - the 'creative'. Many times people cover over their honesty out of physical desire, or out of emotional desire. When we are congruent we are honest from the four levels of our Self. For the noble 'Self' does not allow the wants of one level of our being to create misery for another level. The noble 'Self' always leads us to fulfillment on all four levels. This is relatively rare in human experience in our culture, because we are conditioned and encouraged to seek pure physical gratification, or pure emotional gratification, or pure mental gratification. And this always leads to suffering. To misery. For happiness arises when the integrity of the Whole Self is respected, is met.

I realized in my early twenties, before I found my first significant partner, that a man and I needed to meet on all four levels of my (and his) being in order for me to enter a relationship. That if a man was attracted to me only for my physical, or emotional, or mental stimulation then it could not - for me - be a relationship. This clarity meant that I was single for most of the typical dating years. Yet it meant that, when I finally found a man to be in intimate relationship with, we met in a way that fed my heart, body, mind, and spirit. How nurturing. How inspiring. How delightful. How fulfilling. This is when I began to experience relationship as a way to become more of myself. Because I 'waited' until I met a man who could lure more of me into tangible existence - like a magnet pulling the richness of me out from within my 'shell' and into my active experience of life.

Colin ...

When our experience of life includes the belief that love is in short supply, we may end up in selfish relationships wherein we act out the experience that there's not enough love to go around. And since we all crave love, we become selfish about it. We only exhibit selfish behavior when we fear that our needs will not be met. If there are a million people in a park, you will not see a single person selfishly gasping for more air than they need. Because no one has the perception that there won't be enough fresh air for everyone. But you may witness many people fighting for green space. As in this situation, there may not be enough grass for everyone to be comfortable on.

Because humans have such a distorted relationship with love, most people grow up being manipulated by their parents or some other very influential people in their earlier years through the politics of love. 'If you do this well', or 'If you do what I want ... I will love you more' is a common experience for most people. The opposite of this attitude is that 'If you don't do what I want you to do' or, 'If you're a bad girl or a bad boy ... I will love you less. And you will be punished by being starved of my love and attention.'

What is actually happening in these situations is that these people are not starving us of their loving attention. Rather they are inhibiting us from expressing our love to them. And they are thereby starving us of our connection to love by stopping us from being loving.

Ariole ...

It's so obvious to me as you speak, Colin - like a eureka awareness - why so many people compromise so often in their relationships. They accept the first that comes along and accept whatever disrespect is part of that relationship without knowing how to choose a different partner and how to be different themselves in their relationship. Compromise, as well as dishonesty and its potential for manipulation, have been modeled to most of us simply through standard western parenting.

Look at the classic math equation of a + b = c. If we want a different outcome - a different experience of relationship, a different 'c' - then we need to look at a and b - that which we are endeavoring to create our relationship with. What are the ingredients we are putting into it?

Colin ...

We are selfish when we manipulate. And we are selfless when we treat others with respect. It's that simple. We can treat our lover, our brother and sister, our parents, our children, our neighbor, our colleague and everyone else - and our dog - with respect. All of the time. There is no excuse, ever, for being disrespectful.

Now this really starts with one's self ... Just observe how often our selfish mind is disrespectful to our self. Just notice the negative inner language. And you'll know what I mean.

When you realize this, when you catch yourself being disrespectful with yourself, then pull out your little cheat sheet with the Logical Levels diagram that we've shown you a few pages ago. And ask yourself some open-ended questions like, 'Why did you say that?' 'What do you mean?' 'Who do you think you are, speaking so disrespectfully to me?' 'Who are you?' 'Whose voice is this?' Now really pay attention to whose voice you are hearing. Because it may be someone else's disguised as your own. As you ask yourself these questions you may discover the shocking truth that you have given away your power to the selfish little mind of another person.

This could be your mother, your father, your sibling, teacher or mentor who's mistreated you out of their own pain and suffering. And you must stop this from continuing to happen. So when you ask your inner voice, 'Why did you say that?' you can also continue to state clear boundaries with this voice. Say something like, 'I have a problem when you speak to me like that. And I will no longer hear it. Unless you speak to me with respect, I will remove my attention from you.' That is the action step. To remove your attention from that which is not respectful.

Ariole ...

The etheric is just like the physical - the unseen is just like the seen. The same basic principles apply in metaphysics as in physics. When you invest your attention in something, two things happen. It grows, and you are in an invested relationship with it, with all the effects that that relationship brings about. If you de-invest your energy from something - a person, an activity, an idea - then it no longer grows. You are no longer in relationship with it. And the energy which you had formerly invested in it is now available to you to invest in something / someone else.

It's just like a bank account. Just like real estate. Just like stocks. Just like political and religious systems. What we give our attention to snags us. It grows. And the energy which we've invested in it is not available for something else.

Colin ...

Such as real love. When you say something like, 'My intention is to love you (or life) even more', you feel the power rising up in yourself. You are regaining self consciousness, which is the consciousness of who you are. The true being behind the mind, the body, and the emotions.

Ariole ...

This is what is taught in most schools of Meditation - how to see the mind. How to become aware of the nature of the mind, the nature of the thoughts - even those that typically are silent and 'unheard' by us. When we become able to witness our own mind in this way we are able to clean it out.[1] We regain sovereignty over our mind so that it becomes a tool again - *as it was intended to be -* rather than it our master and us its slave.

---

[1] See the movie "Peaceful Warrior" based on the book <u>Way of the Peaceful Warrior</u> by Dan Millman for an excellent illustration of this.

Connecting to the Divine Lover through the Sovereign Self

C olin ...

It is becoming obvious, I hope, that enjoying a loving and fulfilling relationship requires one to be truthful. And practicing truthfulness and honesty begins with oneself and cannot just be demanded as something practiced by others. It is so common that people blame and complain about their relationships, saying it's the other person's fault. I sincerely hope that with what we are saying here, we are making it absolutely clear that healthy relationships start with one's self.

In this paradigm, it is important that one begins with the proper separation within one self. With separation I mean to separate body from mind from emotions from consciousness, to discover the truth of who I am. Is 'who am I' not the oldest and still unanswered question of humanity?

Let's try to answer this question logically now. When I say, 'I have a body', it becomes clear that I am not my body. Just like when I say, 'I have a car', I cannot be my car. Therefore 'I have a body' cannot mean 'I am my body.' I also talk about my mind. Therefore I am not my mind, I have a mind. I talk about my emotions. Therefore I have emotions, and I cannot be my emotions. I also talk about my spirit. Therefore I have a spirit, but I am not it.

So who am I?

I am an entity, a being, that has a body, that has emotions, that has a mind, and that has a spirit.

Ariole ...

So what we're trying to lead people to is an awareness of the sovereign Self which is not the body, the mind, the emotions, or the spirit. The part of us which can and needs to wholly take responsibility for declaring our well-being - be it in terms of relationship or any other aspect of our life.

When we find within ourselves our sovereign Self, we can no longer be selfish. For the sovereign in us always declares and 'rules' for the good of the whole entity - for the truth and the highest good of the whole system.

This is an entirely different way of being in relationship. It is what we might call … 'mature'. For in all the ways that so many of us typically behave selfishly in relationship, we are being immature. We are behaving as children cut off from the source, cut off from true, infinite and boundless love. When we live in scarcity, we are behaving as if we are cut off from the divine.

So connecting with our sovereign is connecting with the divine.

Colin …

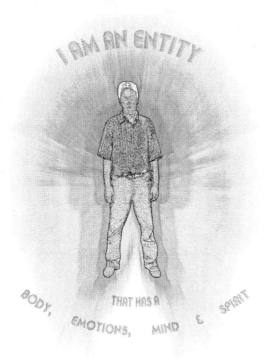

Seeing the divine in each other is the easy way - the easy process - the effortless path to building and main-taining life-long, loving and fulfilling relationships. Most people are limited in their perception by the physical. That is, they are conditioned to only perceive life through their five senses. So they're attracted on a physical level. They get involved sexually. This creates an emotion. They don't know how to deal with it intelligently. And because they're not connected with the divine they are subjected to the fear of death and dying. Yet the divine is their connection to love. And being connected only to the mortal, physical self, their relationship suffocates ... in the selfish fear of death.

The remedy to this is very, very simple. Acknowledge the beauty that you see in the person who is in front of you now. Acknowledge their beauty in a way that is appropriate according to the relationship that you have with that person. When we acknowledge what is beautiful, we get beyond our prejudices. We transcend the small, critical, judgmental voice that can only see the negative or the perceived imperfection in the creation that is the other person.

Ariole ...

Not everyone will appreciate us in the short term for seeing their divinity. Some will be relieved by it, as if they have waited all their life to be recognized for the inner joy and brilliance and radiance that they truly are.

For in seeing the divinity in someone we are calling it forth from them. If they perceive themselves as contrary to this - as undeserving of love, for instance, as a result of a misperception of guilt and shame arising from a wound - then they may reject our seeing the divinity in them. They may push us away, trying to reiterate and prove their unworthiness of love - of God.

What we do then is simply remain sensitive to them, seeing the truth which is their divinity, the god / love in them. We see their truth, their love, while demanding nothing.

With those who are awakened by our recognition of their divinity, we simply continue to see the truth in them, thus accelerating their embodying it. In so doing they shed their former illusion of their lovelessness. We assist them, simply by witnessing their divinity, to quicken themselves to truth. To being love.

Love is the only truth. We are all love. In fact, we are nothing other than love. What confuses life - and relationships - is that we forget. We become lured by a misperception that we are guilty … simply for existing. That we are sinful for being. That the co-creative process, of which we were born, is somehow sinful. And so we 'hide'. We believe, on a level of perception so unconscious to us, that if we remain small and 'godless', then this ultimate sin might go unnoticed.

The truth is so far from this. In fact, it is 180° 'rotated' in relation to it. It is 'upside down'.

The truth is that we are love. And a healthy relationship, a soulful relationship, a growth-oriented relationship, will naturally and consistently return us to this truth. That we are love. That we always have been love. That everyone else is love. We're just a wounded species which has forgotten this.

Colin ...

Why not give others the opportunity to be kind and loving when they express their desire to be so? How often do we turn down other people's kind gestures? Saying, 'This is not necessary.' 'Don't fuss about it.' So one way to be more loving is to grant other people the opportunity to express more love. Receive a compliment graciously. Don't make it smaller. Receive the flowers and say, 'Thank you.' Instead of, 'You didn't have to.'

Ariole ...

Yes, it's amazing ... all the little ways that we stunt each other's love. All the ways that we, barely visibly, diminish the presence of love in human society.

Colin ...

Do you ever plant a rosebush and, as it starts to grow and blossom, say to it, 'Oh, don't bother. That's not necessary. No thank you?' Of course you don't. So let's treat other people just like we would treat a beautiful, delicate rose bush with all its petals and thorns.

People are no different. We all have petals, and thorns. And they are there for a good reason. When we accept this, and cultivate our 'rose bush', we're well on our way to unlocking the secret to a fulfilling love relationship.

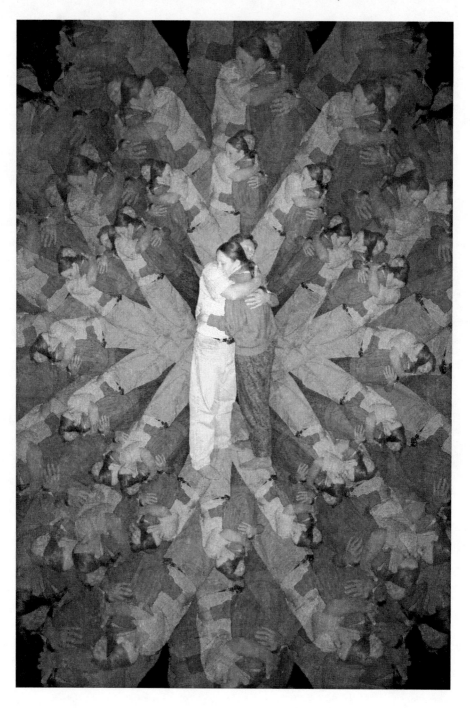

Cultivating your 'Rose Bush'

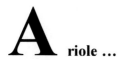

A riole ...

A practice which Colin introduced to our relationship in its early months was so effective in cultivating our rose bush. (We actually planted a rose bush during our wedding ceremony and we gave each of our guests a tiny rose bush.)

At night, as we lay in bed, we would take as long as we needed for a simple conversation. One person would begin. The other would simply listen, saying nothing. When they were complete, the second person would begin and the first person would listen, silently.

The framework of this simple conversation was always the same. There were the beginnings of two sentences. Each night our endings to these two sentences would evolve.

'I am grateful for ... '

'I forgive you for ... '

This little exercise lay the groundwork for us to be truthful with each other - grateful, and forgiving, expressing clearly what we wished might be different while being thankful for what we had in each other. Our respect for each other deepened quantumly each and every time we practiced this 'exercise'.

After a year or so we found that we didn't need it anymore. It had contributed so much to creating a solid groundwork of respect and clear, honest communication in our relationship. I highly recommend this simple, powerful exercise to any couple who wants to 'get it right'. Gratitude and forgiveness are two key ingredients in this recipe for an honest relationship that is built on respect, truthfulness, and trust.

Colin ...

When you practice this exercise you will soon realize its inherent benefit - that nothing remains hidden. If you're not in a relationship or your partner doesn't want to participate, then do this on your own. Speak to yourself. 'This is what I'm grateful for about me. And this is what I forgive myself for.' It's very powerful. It can save your life.

Ariole ...

Yes. When we practice this exercise, honestly, it is impossible for resentments to build up. And accumulated resentments are the poison of most relationships.

Colin ...

So true. Because ... let's say you practice this exercise with your partner. And then one day you say to your partner, 'Well, I'm going to leave you now because this or that is wrong about you or us.' Then your partner has every right to say to you, 'How come you never brought it up? How come you never had the courage to say it when we talked about gratitude and forgiveness?' Then you must face yourself. And ask, 'How could I have been so dishonest? With myself, and with my lover? How come I never had the courage to address the fact? What can I do now to regain my self-respect?'

Ariole ...

What we're seeking - in entering into and being in relationship - is to cultivate so much truthfulness in ourselves that we cannot accept a new relationship that doesn't hold the premise of truthfulness. We cannot accept the continuation of a relationship that doesn't hold the premise of truthfulness. In being fearless of 'death' - realizing that the divine is ephemeral, eternal - we are unafraid to be strong in our choices. Unwilling to allow ourselves to enter into or continue in relationships which do not demonstrate that they are capable of truth.

Spiritual Consciousness - Our Sixth Sense

C olin ...

What leads us to this kind of truth is our sixth sense. A sense which is not of our physical body. A sense which we generally refer to as 'intuition'.

Ariole ...

Yes. In **HeartSong Matchmaking**™, and in all of our Coaching, Healing, and Learning sessions with clients, we support them - to the degree that they invite us and allow us to - to access their intuition. To actually begin to live by it. To learn to recognize it, trust it, heed it and strengthen it such that it becomes their greatest consultant, their greatest advisor, their greatest guide, their greatest ally. Intuition is like a muscle. It becomes stronger with use. And Spirit gives us more intuitive guidance as we use what we are given. Our life, in essence, thus turns inside out as we begin to listen to the great voice 'within' rather than deferring so much of our power to the voices and influences without.

Colin ...

There seems to be increased interest in learning about intuition. Clients often ask what it is, how to recognize it, where to feel it, where it comes from, and what to do about it. Intuition arises from a particular level of consciousness. There are four levels of consciousness. Physical consciousness, emotional consciousness, mental consciousness, and spiritual consciousness.

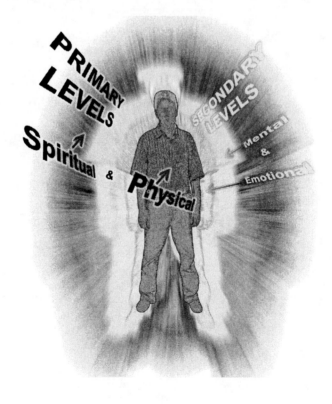

Colin ...

Intuition is a function of the fourth level of consciousness. It arises from our spiritual self. Intuition is something we can equate to our inner knowing - our hunches, generally known as our 'gut feeling'. When we begin to awaken to our higher levels of consciousness we become increasingly aware of our intuition - our gut sense. In the beginning we notice it and it becomes a challenge to have the courage to follow it - to act on it. Why? Because the level of consciousness that is below spiritual consciousness - mental consciousness - produces the rational thinking that we experience as self doubt. So what happens in practical terms is that our true self informs us and a function of consciousness at a lower level questions it and thereby sabotages our ability to do the right thing.

Ariole ...

So in effect, following our intuition more frequently - and thus strengthening our 'intuition muscle' - effectively transfers our 'god' - the great advisor that we worship - from our rational mind to our intuition.

This is **so important** because it is our intuition - not our rational mind - which can see the path(s) of greatest growth and opportunity for us. Our rational thinking is based upon what we already know, in this lifetime, as 'information'. Our intuition has access to all Knowing. It is a tap into All Knowing.

Our intuition is like a bird, flying high above us, able to see all that is around us - including present and future possibility. It can 'see' ... where the waters flow smoothly, and where there are boulders, obstacles, and debris in our future way. It guides us, painlessly and effortlessly, into constant *flow*.

Perhaps the reason many people fear their intuition prior to discovering its grace, benevolence, and incredible expediency is that it *always* guides us into new territories of growth. It is spirit. It is of Spirit. Its 'job' is to grow us. To lead us out of our limitations, our small beliefs and actions, into the true splendour of who we are and who we can become.[1]

Colin ...

The true purpose of the mental consciousness is to process, through logical thinking, the intuitive impulses. And here is where most people create problems in their lives. They use the faculties of mind in rational ways rather than in logical ways. Rational thinking leads to false conclusions that are based on pride and prejudice. Pride and prejudice leads to shame and guilt. And thus a person

---

[1] See also <u>Birds' Eye View - A Travel Guide to the Universe</u> by Ariole K. Alei.

who processes his or her life experiences through rational thinking remains stuck in the lower levels of consciousness. David Hawkins MD, a brilliant healer, researcher and writer describes the levels of consciousness in his ground-breaking book <u>Power versus Force</u>. According to Hawkins, it is in the lower levels of consciousness that humans force themselves upon others with their shame, guilt, fear, anger, desire, and false pride. All of these levels of mind and emotions arise out of rational thinking. Such as, 'I can't marry her because she's of a different faith.' 'I am too young or too old, too thin or too fat, too rich or too poor, not educated enough, etcetera.'

So the mind basically has these two functions.

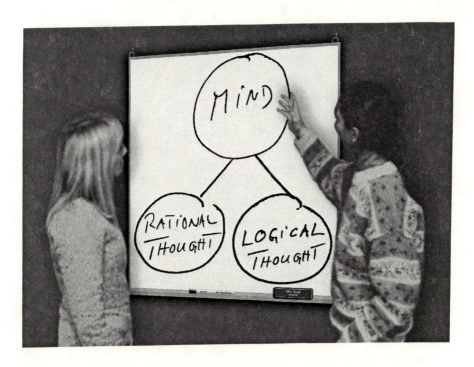

Colin ...

The purpose of mental consciousness is to process, through a logical application, the information received from above - the intuition.

For example, one might have the intuitive hunch to call uncle Bob.

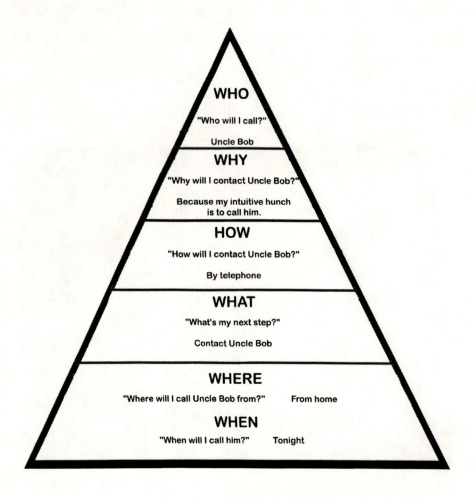

The intuitive hunch says, 'call uncle Bob.' If a person is accustomed to processing thought in a rational way, the mind might respond, 'It's too expensive to call, because he lives at the other end of the world.' At that point, the spiritual impulse might be braked and killed off by a personal prejudice that comes out of the conditioned mind saying, 'It's too expensive. I can't afford it.'

A logical process following the intuitive hunch 'Call uncle Bob' might be, 'How can I get to a phone? Where's the nearest phone and my calling card?' So the logical thinker who has the courage to take pure practical action on his or her intuitive guidance never doubts the 'order' that comes from above. He or she gets to the phone, calls uncle Bob at the other side of the world, and uncle Bob says, 'I'm so glad to hear from you. I just won the lottery. And I can't find your address to send you a cheque!'

Ariole ...

Yes. Even when the intuitive impulse or 'order' seems simple, small, inconsequential, when we **follow it** we discover that it has led us to somewhere very magical. In my experience this is true each and every time. We cannot see the great mysteries which surround us, always, in every moment, from the place of a human who believes that she or he is 'small'. A person who believes that all that exists is what can be measured through the five human 'outer' senses. The intuition is here to awaken us beyond that. To awaken us, in its gentle yet irrevocable way, to all that we *forgot when we were born.*

What's more, when we begin to trust the 'orders that come from above', we discover that we are trusting a higher level of our own Self. And through it, a higher level of All That Is. Intuition is transportable. And it costs nothing. Everyone has access to it. We are all wired into it even though many, many of us have rusty, old, unused wires. We *all* have **direct access** to the Divine - call it what you will - through our own internal 'telephone', our own intuition link.[2]

---

2 See also <u>Awakening Instinct - the true feminine principle</u> by Ariole K. Alei.

The Wise Lovers

C olin ...

All good books contain a secret. And if there was one secret to creating and enjoying a fulfilling love relationship, it is this: Abandon rational thought. Listen to and act on your intuition. Process this information logically. Be loving and respectful.

Rational thinking is the mother of death in a potentially loving and fulfilling relationship. Sooner or later, when the first wave of romance comes to a lull, the ordinary person becomes disenchanted, frustrated, possibly even angry because the other person no longer 'measures up'. Measures up to what? Not measuring up to a higher expectation which is based on rational thought. Such as, 'She should be more available for sex.' This judgement is based on what? It is an idea that is rooted in past experience. It requires the rational mind to compare the current status to a historical fact. Do you see the dilemma? The rational thinker is caught in a trap of duality. Rational thinking requires at least two points of reference, this and that. It is selfish and devoid of love and respect.

Ariole ...

In duality we experience separation, or the anticipation of separation which, because we focus on it, naturally creates or attracts or magnetically draws separation towards us. We create what we focus on. The mind is this potent, this powerful, this strong. We are doing this all the time, every one of us.[1] Yet because we don't culturally validate this as being 'real' - because we cannot measure and see brain waves, how they set out and travel in the 'world', what they speak to and dialogue with, and what they bring 'home' - we do not believe that **we are this powerful**. We are doing this all the time, now. When we wake up to this - when we realize what we are doing with our mind - we enter a unique, 'new' position of *choosing what we want to create and attract with the power of our thoughts.* With what we choose to focus our mind upon. Our mind is like the sun, shining on a reflective surface. Given enough 'time' it creates fire. Where did this fire come from? The heat of the sun. The heat of the *mind.* The heat of our mind creates whatever it focuses on for enough 'time'. Our mind is like the sun creating fire. This is a natural principle. It is true. It is real. It works even if we do not realize it. The sun creates fire - when it shines on a reflective object for enough 'time' - even if it is not consciously intending to.

---

[1] See the movie "The Secret" for an excellent elucidation of this.

Spirit - The Source of Self

Colin ...

Just like there is only one sun, there is only one thing to do: What intuition tells us through our gut knowing. Following our intuition by taking pure practical action keeps us from the dreadful experience of separation and empowers us to be one with the source of love. Spirit. Love and oneness is what everyone seeks.

When we consciously climb the Mountain of Life we reduce our dualistic thinking, and as we reach higher and higher levels we experience fewer emotional pendulum swings. Ultimately, we reach the true point of oneness and pure being.

Ariole ...

When you said, "We reduce our ..." I heard in my mind, 'We reduce our emissions!' As we awaken we become more and more co-creative with Source, and often we find ourselves in the midst of cosmic laughter - cosmic jokes! As you continued speaking I realized that the 'emissions' analogy is true! (Cosmic jokes always are!!) As we climb higher on the Mountain of Life we do have less 'emissions'! We have less 'baggage'. We have less guck in us. We are polluting less.

We travel lighter ...

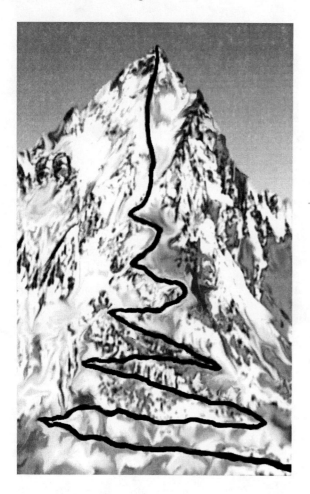

This image illustrates this so well. The higher we rise, the degree of duality decreases. There are fewer and fewer pendulum 'swings' - less and less duality. So it becomes obvious that the peak is the point of Oneness - a place of no duality.

It's fascinating how these metaphors are always so powerful, and so incredibly 'more real than real'.

Ascending the Mountain Together
- New Paradigm Lovers

C olin ...

What can you, the reader, do now that you've come to the end of this book? Where do you go from here? Let's summarize: Climbing the Mountain of Life is as simple as 1 – 2 – 3.

Step #1: Let your intuition lead you up. The mountain represents consciousness. And you already are in the process of evolving consciously. So just surrender to the process and let it happen. *Learn how to 'get out of your own way.'*

Step #2: Process your intuitive knowing, your hunches, your gut sense, with the logical thinking process.

Step #3: Don't make a move until you know the truth. You discover the truth by asking Logical Level questions until you are satisfied with what you've found. Which can only be the truth. Most people make the mistake of not asking enough logical questions. They thereby end up frustrated and angry due to a process known as 'incomplete communication'. They end up spinning in circles or shutting the door rather than moving forward. Don't move until you know the truth. Then, take powerful, pure practical action steps.

Being There - Now

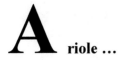

A riole ...

Notice yourself climbing the Mountain with your chosen partner. Become aware ... how easy it has become ... to ascend your Mountain as you have learned and practiced how to ask Logical Levels questions. 'Where am I?' 'Where is my next step?' 'What is it?' 'What do I need?' 'What do I need to let go of?'

Notice that the higher you ascend this Mountain the less baggage you are carrying. This is a paradox. To climb higher you must let go the baggage. In climbing, your former baggage falls away from you.

Where is your partner? Notice how you have become each other's allies. How you have learned to believe in each other, to support each other, to challenge each other to live your full capabilities. Notice how you lovingly challenge each other when it is the other who holds the light of courage for you. Notice what it feels like to have your partner believe in you so deeply and profoundly.

Look back. Look back down the Mountain to the path you have traveled. Notice how far you have come. Notice how you have changed, how you have transformed. What is different about you now? How do you feel about yourself? How do you relate to the Mountain? What has changed in your belief about your capabilities? What have you already demonstrated that you can do - by doing it? How has your relationship with your partner transformed? What is it like for you to truly have an ally - and to be an ally? What is it like to climb the Mountain together?

Take a moment and celebrate all the plateaus that you have already reached. Did you rush through them? Take an extra moment now to reflect upon, savour, and congratulate yourself for all that you have achieved in terms of transformation, growth, and ascension of the Mountain. How far are you up the Mountain? Does it get easier or more challenging as you ascend? Take a few moments to rest, to celebrate - alone and/or with your partner. And when you feel ready ... continue with your ascension!

...

You are an amazing being.

Your Mountain is a beautiful and wondrous Mountain.

Celebrate your Mountain. Celebrate your self. Celebrate your Life.

This is a joyous journey. A magical journey. A remarkable opportunity. Be grateful for this Mountain. Be grateful for your partner.

Be grateful for yourself.

Thank Life.

...

Thank You.

♥ Colin and Ariole

Last Chapter – True Love
- Making a Difference

 Soul Searching Exercise

Please write the Final Chapter of this book by reflecting upon *your response* … to this question …

Who else benefits when I love more?

If you feel drawn to, submit your Final Chapter to us at info@veraxis.net. With your consent you may see your written expression of more love in this world in print on our websites! Visit us at www.veraxis.net and www.HeartSongSolutions.ca.

Share your vision of a loving planet - one in which men and women cherish and respect each other! Imagine … What might this be like?

Appendix

Daily Reflections
- **Pure Practical Action**
- *Your Next Steps*

Create a journal - or simply use these pages as a guide to ask yourself - daily - the following questions. Notice how quickly your life changes for the better as you give *daily attention* to yourself, to your partner or desired partner, to your mountain, to Life.

Enjoy your journey!

And remember, we are here to assist you, to guide you if you wish to receive our support. See the **HeartSong** section at the end of the Appendix!

For Singles

Ask yourself these Logical Levels questions …

Where am I on the mountain? Look at the picture below.
What does my intuition tell me? Where am I now?

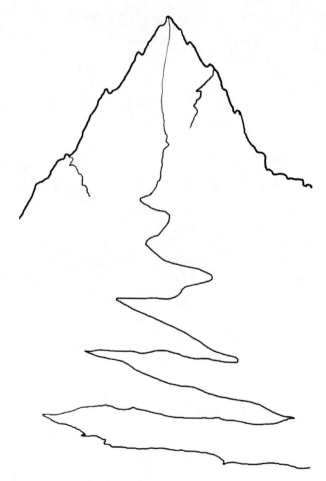

Where do I want to go next?

How might I get there?

With whom?

How will I know when I'm there?

What must I stop doing and thinking so I can further ascend my mountain?

What else must change?

What might it be like to reach the next level?
>What might I see? Hear? Feel? Taste? Smell?

When am I going to make the next move up?

What new skills must I acquire?

Is my health and level of fitness good enough to reach the top of the mountain? If not, what can I do about it?

Are my finances and my financial blueprint - my inner financial thermostat - sufficient to fund the next expedition?

What are the exact attributes of my ideal climbing partner?

Who else benefits when I consciously and actively move towards the top of my mountain? Who benefits when I love more?

For Couples

Ask yourself these Logical Levels questions …

Where am I on the mountain? Where is my partner? What does our intuition tell us? Where are we now?

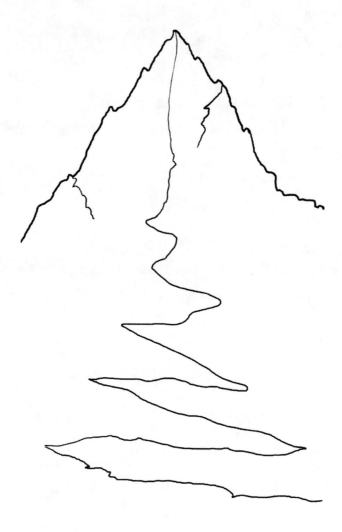

Where do we want to go next?

How might we get there?

How can we help each other rise to the next higher plateau?

How can we become stronger allies as climbing partners?

What must we stop doing and thinking?

What else must change?

What might it be like to reach the next level?
>What might we see? Hear? Feel? Taste? Smell?

When are we going to make the next move up?

Which new skills must we acquire?

Is our health and level of fitness good enough to reach the next level? If not, what can we do about it?

Are our finances and our financial blueprint - our inner financial thermostat - sufficient to fund the next expedition?

How can we create more oneness between us?

Who else benefits when we consciously and actively move towards the top of our mountain? When we *love more?*

Bibliography

Ariole K. Alei, *Awakening Instinct - the true feminine principle / Running the Gauntlet – navigating our way to our fully embodied potential / Windows Through Time - a 'possible evolution story'*, HeartSong Solutions, Vancouver Canada, 2006

Ariole K. Alei, *Birds' Eye View - A Travel Guide to the Universe*, HeartSong Solutions, Vancouver Canada, 2006

Barry Long, *To Man In Truth*, Barry Long Books, London England, 1999

Barry Long, *To Woman In Love*, Barry Long Books, London England, 1994

Colin Hillstrom, *When A Man Really Loves A Woman*, HeartSong Solutions, Vancouver Canada, 2006

Colin Hillstrom, *Your 2ⁿᵈ Life - How to Live the Life You Always Wanted*, HeartSong Solutions, Vancouver Canada, 2006

Dan Brown, *The Da Vinci Code,* Doubleday, USA, 2003

Dan Millman, *The Life You Were Born To Live*, HJ Kramer Inc, Tiburon CA USA, 1993

David Hawkins, *Power vs. Force*, Hay House, Inc., Carlsbad CA USA, 1995

Don Miguel Ruiz, *The Mastery of Love*, Amber-Allen Publishing, Inc., San Rafael CA USA, 1999

Gary Zukav, *The Seat of the Soul*, Fireside, New York USA, 1989

Harvey and Marilyn Diamond, *Fit for Life*, Warner Books, USA, 1987

Raffi Cavoukian and Sharna Olfman, *Child Honouring: How to Turn This World Around,* www.raffinews.com, 2006

Ariole's Story

I was born into a respectful, intelligent, caring, and integrated family in all outwardly observable ways. In my parents' generation, everyone was university educated, having created more in terms of quality of life and affluence than the generation before them.

Our family was societally engaged, participating as patrons to the arts, active voters (though not politically opinionated), and contributing professionals, neighbors, mentors, and volunteers.

In many ways we were viewed as a model family. I felt energized and respected by this as, for the most part, it was true.

My grandfather and my second cousin both fought in the war. For my grandfather, it was the First World War; for my second cousin, it was the Second. Although I was not yet born to witness these wars and their horrors directly, I did experience them. The trauma which each of these men experienced was, ultimately, passed on to me.

It was much later, when I had laid the foundation for remembering and healing the deep wounds of sexual and, on one occasion, ritual abuse, that I had 'flashes'. Flashes in which I remembered the energy of my perpetrators at the moments of violation. In these flashes, I also saw war. I saw that the terror and trauma which these men experienced *and did not integrate, heal, and resolve* - in moments of overwhelm - and advantage - they put this terror out on me.

I was always a 'spiritually connected' child. I spent a lot of time alone in nature. I 'scribed poetry', created many works of art with my hands, communed with wild creatures, reveled under the moonlit sky. And I danced. (See www.sharonwehnerdance.com – Ariole's birth name and dance company.) I danced from the age of seven in what quickly revealed itself to me as a safe haven. A world in which reality and mystery were blurred - so inextricably woven that I could discover my 'true' self amidst the rubble and confusion (albeit forgotten then by me) of the abuse. It was a confusing reality, my life. So much richness and love … and hidden violation. Betrayal. Breech of trust.

I learned - not because anyone told me this directly - how to keep a hidden secret.

I had a motto when I was young, that, 'I trust people until they give me a reason to do otherwise.' I was incredibly trusting considering the betrayal which I had repeatedly experienced. The spirit is *so* wise, and the soul so forgiving and resilient.

I was a successful, capable person in so many ways. From the outside, without the 'eyes' necessary to spot the effects of abuse, I appeared to be a sterling child. I was adept in so many things, excelling in virtually everything I attempted or desired. In a way my life was magic.

When I reached my early twenties the deep, hidden waters began to break loose. The terror which was culturally supported to go unseen, ignored … it could no longer be contained. To evolve as the *human being that I am* it was time for the abuse to be remembered - for me to be set free.

I was twenty-eight when I first touched a man sexually. I had had ten boyfriends prior to that, each of whom - thanks to my incredible guidance and ability to call respectful young men to me - did not force themselves beyond my wishes.

The truth was, I was frozen. I would wonder - as if 'I' was distant, existing 'away from' my body - why I didn't feel *anything* when they touched me. And why … I seemed to have no desire.

It wasn't until the right moment - a safe man, sufficient inner awakening stirring within myself, sufficient maturity and psychological fortitude to ride the upcoming waves and storm - that I actually made love with a man. I was twenty-eight. And I was petrified.

This event - what for many women much younger than I is a joyous, rapturous, and life-cherishing moment - was the unleashing of a wild tiger. I entered therapy. My knee and hand broke in order to create a gestalt in my life. I could not work as a professional dancer, at least for some time, as my body healed *and my spirit healed.* As I perceived it then, my body, in all its wisdom, generosity and grace, acquiesced itself that my heart might heal.

I went through three major healing spirals over the next decade, each of them awakening me deeper and deeper to my authentic self. To the spirit within me.

One of the awarenesses, the observations which absolutely spellbound me, was how ... it's not the traumatic event itself that creates the changes in one's life. The event happens, and it's done. It is the decisions, the beliefs, the patterns of mind and heart and body which are 'decided' as a result of it that then permeate like tiny fingers throughout every aspect of one's life. And so the healing is not merely the healing of 'the event'. It is the healing of who we have become as a result of it. It is the rediscovering of who we are beneath it - who we were before it - and who we are now, beyond it.

I was thirty-four when I entered my first serious relationship.

I was forty when I married for the first time.

I realized, in the course of my healing, that I chose the wound of incest. I remember precisely the series of moments before incarnating into this lifetime when I chose this event. I chose it in order to be effective in my work here - my purpose in incarnating in this lifetime. I realized that, in order for others to allow me to assist them in their healing and their awakening - they would need to trust me. And to trust me with the depths of their anguish, and their sorrow, they would need to know that I understood.

How could I understand, to the depth that they required of me in order to trust me with their selves - if I didn't understand, *through experience,* the perils of human suffering? The confusion and turmoil of human dynamics?

The only way they would let me in to do what I came here to do, would be for me to live an aspect of what they have lived. Belly to belly, unconscious mind to deep unconscious mind, they would trust me if I *knew.*

This recognition held a context in which I could deeply and profoundly heal. And still, I knew within me that my healing would not be complete without living an aspect of it with a man. That being with a man, in a healthy and a fearless way, was necessary to complete my healing. I could not do it all 'alone'.

When I met Colin I was blown away by his philosophy of relationship. His understanding of the dynamics of human intimate relationships. And his vision of the healing of the planet *through* the healing of the man / woman relationship.

I was so inspired when he first conveyed his philosophy to me ... that a 'man' perceived this. Knew this. Spoke of this. Espoused this.

I wondered ... could he actually live it, too?

I felt massive fear when I first met Colin. I knew fear well enough through many experiences which my spirit and my intuition had led me into and guided me through, to recognize the distinction between fear which is a signal of danger - a message to 'flee' ... and fear which is a signal ... of tremendous near future personal growth. My fear 'of Colin' was the latter. Immediately when I recognized this, I knew. His presence in my life would 'hold the space' for boundless growth for me.

When I 'looked in' to see if I could sense how long our relationship would endure for ... I could not see a limit. What I did see was that ... he had the capacity to hold the space for me to self actualize - to become, on this planet, in this flesh, the enormity of Light which I am here to be.

To me, this is a model of true relationship - spiritual relationship, sacred relationship. Preparing ourselves through healing, growing, and awakening to be ready for - and to attract - the partner who will hold the space for us to burst forth from our invisible shells and radiate into Life.

Ultimately, relationship *is* Life. In Life, no thing is independent or stands alone. We all support each other. This is the nature of symbiosis, of systems, of living systems. We all exist to nurture and to feed each other in the most inspiring and healthy ways.

It is my hope that, with the inspiration, learning, and experience that we share with you, you too may find - and keep - the love of your dreams. The man or woman who calls forth from within you the gems and inner riches that you perhaps didn't even know were there.

For we are all radiant beings of Light, many of us tarnished and in disbelief of this wondrous fact. And as we see in each other this radiant glory - and in its Light, as we 'forgive' what we have done and said in 'past' as a remnant of our slumber and our innocence - we truly will become the 'children of God'. The enlightened race.

Colin's Story
- "PAPA WAS A ROLLING STONE"

I began studying and applying fundamental health principles around 1987 when, at the age of twenty-eight, my health was in a mess.

Today, at the age of forty-seven, people generally don't believe that it is possible that a man who started on a path of serious drinking and smoking at the age of nine can look ten or more years younger than he is. How is this possible?

The answer is NATURAL HEALTH.

Back at the age of twenty-eight I had to face a choice of how to deal with chronic bronchitis. While I was still enjoying alcohol, tobacco, coffee, meat and sweets in large amounts, I was getting annoyed at how my ailing respiratory system was getting in the way of my pleasures!

There were two factors which steered me in the direction of natural health.

One - I was born and raised in Germany with the attitude that you only use pharmaceuticals if you absolutely have to, and two - a brother-in-law had told me about his mother's miraculous experience (she had been battling terminal cancer) with a wheatgrass and raw food therapy at the Hippocrates Health Institute.

I soon found myself in a new job and out of town training during which I could provide for myself in a hotel room for three weeks. Prior to leaving for this trip I decided to drop a fourth year accounting course (Accounting Theory, which is as stimulating as watching a cow chew grass for hours). Returning the textbook at the university bookstore, a book on an entirely new subject fell into my hands ... Fit For Life by Harvey Diamond.

Within three weeks of applying the principles of "Natural Hygiene" as they were described by Dr. Diamond, my excess weight started to peel-off rather quickly. I was more then pleased. Natural healing had caught my interest.

Next, I read Dr. Ann Wigmore's books about wheatgrass, sprouting and raw food diets. Within a couple of months my kitchen had turned into a green room. Wheatgrass, oatgrass, alfalfa sprouts, radish sprouts, clover sprouts, sunflower greens and buckwheat greens were decorating the inner landscape of my home.

I was getting healthier. My sleep was amazingly light and restful. But there was another a problem. While I was getting healthier I was often getting sick, even violently ill. How could this be?

The issue was that while I had changed my diet, I hadn't quit drinking and smoking. My body was reacting violently to new toxins because it had become clearer inside. I finally had a severe case of pneumonia. While the doctors were searching for effective antibiotics, an older patient died next to me in his hospital bed. For the first time in my life I feared death.

I made a resolution to completely change my lifestyle and become clear, clean, and pure inside. At that time I could still only relate this concept to my physical body. Three months later I and my family relocated from south-western Ontario to super natural British Columbia.

Vancouver's fresh air and mountain trails, organic food, wheatgrass, sprouts and aphanezomenon flos aqua (Super Blue Green Algae® harvested by Cell Tech Inc,[1]) were the best therapy for me.

---

[1] Visit www.HealthyFutures.net/ColinHillstrom for FREE Nutrition Courses and other information.

I did not touch alcohol or cigarettes for almost five years and thrived on a vegan diet. My lungs recuperated so well that I never had a cold or flu again. I believe that the Super Blue Green Algae™ played a significant role in this for two reasons. Energetically speaking, each food has a certain signature, meaning it nourishes a specific aspect of our physiology and anatomy. Algae are the respiratory system of the earth and therefore contribute special healing energy to our respiratory system. Furthermore, the blue green colour spectrum of the Super Blue Green Algae™ I believe nourished my heart chakra and my throat chakra, as well as the thymus chakra which is located between these two.

When I moved to Vancouver in 1990 I did not understand energy at all. But I had been sharing my nutritional knowledge with many others during the two years prior and enjoyed helping others with their health. While I was working for Revenue Canada as a Tax Interpretations Officer and a Seminar Leader to educate the public on the emerging GST, I started taking certificate courses at Wild Rose College in Iridology and Applied Kinesiology. This connected me with other healers. I soon started practicing part-time as an Iridologist and Nutritionist and I joined the Board of the BC Holistic Healers Association.

Through the monthly Board meetings I was introduced to the practice of meditation which would eventually become a pillar of my personal spiritual practice.

"Papa Was A Rolling Stone" really is the story of a man who used to be a restless man. Equipped with a typical ADD/ADHD type brain, my bi-polar behavior had left a trail marked by frequent relocations, job changes and business start-ups, unfinished projects, divorce, self-indulgence, self-pity, grandiosity, rage, anger, infidelities and depression.

It was through my passion for natural healing that I gradually transformed the tyrant, the weakling, the sadist, the masochist, the manipulator and the addict into a mature man.

Deepak Chopra, Stuart Wilde, Chris Griscom, Dan Millman, John Randolph Price, Neil Donald Walsh, Louise L. Hay, Robert Michael Kaplan, Robert Moore & Douglas Gillette, Jacob Lieberman, Gary Zukav, Osho, Stephen Covey and in particular Barry Long have illuminated my life-path through their spiritual teachings. Being a spiritual seeker has helped me to see what was wrong with me and take 'right' action.

When I met my second and present wife in 1999 I was sufficiently still inside to hold the space for Ariole to accelerate her sexual healing. I soon discovered that her process sped-up my own healing. When I discovered in 2001 through a medical diagnosis that I had a severe case of ADD/ADHD, I could immediately trace back my emotional instability and suicidal thoughts to their root cause. At this time I had sufficient experience with self-healing that I could acknowledge, accept and act in virtually 'no time'.

The subsequent discovery of Dr. Robert Moore's model of the Jungian Four Archetypes in <u>King, Warrior, Magician, Lover</u> helped me to 're-wire' my brain almost instantly.

But it is the idea and the teaching of spiritual relationship (Gary Zukav in <u>Seat Of The Soul</u>), and the commitment to honesty and openness between Man and Woman (Barry Long in <u>Making Love</u>) that have influenced my life more than anything else.

There is no end to our growing, to our unfolding, to our loving. I fully acknowledge that certain layers had to be peeled off before I could hear the words of the masters. When I look back to who I once was, I rejoice. Because I am constantly changing, I know that everyone else can. The potential for loving and being more is present at all times in every man and woman and child.

Today, the greatest gift to me is that I can look beyond people's masks and recognize their essence, and see 'what is'…

'What is' is always beautiful, still, deep and endless.

Infinite, immortal, eternal, universal…

Like all of us.

Excerpts from Our Other Books

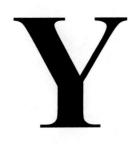 OUR 2ND LIFE
How to Live the Life You Always Wanted
* Book, CD, and Manual *

by Colin Hillstrom

Intro to Y2L – "Your 2nd Life"

In the summer of 2001 I came across an article by the late Robert DeRopp called "The Mastergame". What immediately intrigued me about it was the idea that one should choose a game worth playing and play it with all one's courage, and that one should not allow oneself to be distracted or discouraged by the negative emotions of those who are closest - our family and friends.

Having experienced the detrimental influence of family and friends myself, it was easy for me to feel that Mr. DeRopp's theory was very valid. I struggled though with the concept of picking a particular game. What if my choice would be wrong? What if my imagination were to lead me down the wrong path? I had read in the liner notes of Elton John's milestone album "Goodbye Yellow Brick Road" that "… Bernie Taupin had experienced the high life of which he had dreamed and seemingly found it less satisfactory."

Why is it that many personal growth gospels teach that you must use the imagination of your mind in order to create success? Isn't this what Mr. Taupin had so successfully done? He imagined success and he successfully manifested this vision. How about John Lennon? Why had he retreated from the 'high life' before his passing? (Recommendation: watch the movie "The Two Of Us" about an imaginary one day encounter of Paul McCartney and John Lennon in John's New York apartment in 1976.)

In my life I have met many individuals with above average career, business and financial success. I grew up in an environment of successful entrepreneurs and I have witnessed predominantly disharmonious marriages, addictions, depression, diseases, broken families and broken dreams.

In 47 years I have encountered only one family where the first marriage was still vibrant, loving and harmonious, where the lifestyle was second to none, health was good, and all five children and grandchildren still loved to play with the old folks.

This is astonishing. One family in how many?

What about all the 'winners' I knew who had picked their games, taken their risks, dreamed and lived their dreams, and succeeded financially yet had ended up with shattered lives?

Something must be missing in the popular formulas for success, I thought. Mr. DeRopp's idea of the "Mastergame" still intrigued me and I kept looking. I finally traced down a copy of his book The Mastergame which had been a huge hit in the 60's. Fortunately, the book had been recently reprinted.

In his Conclusion to The Mastergame, Mr. DeRopp describes the idea of "the second life". What he is saying is that our life has four segments: (1) in utero, (2) growing up, (3) building a career and raising a family, and (4) enjoying our life after the children are mature and are independently building their own phase '(3)'.

It is the 4th phase, which can stretch from the age of 50 to 100, which is our second life. The missing link for most people in making this theory real is what I call 'perfect life balance'. Our ability to enjoy our 'Golden Years' is directly related to how successfully we have managed phases two and three of our life.

In my experience, the people who I had grown up with had failed to pay equal attention to all areas of their life. The error they had made was in neglecting the key areas of health, love, mentoring, and character development.

As a result, despite their financial prosperity, their troubled marriages, problematic children, and ill health had bankrupted their overall lives and had denied them the enjoyment of their second life.

You don't have to duplicate their errors and thus their fate.

It's up to you.

Yes, you can have it all. Learn how, and commit to improving your *overall* game.

<u>Your 2nd Life – How To Live The Life You Always Wanted</u> addresses all the key life areas with clarity and authority.

Written from both my personal and professional experience, this program will lead you through essays, exercises, and a guided 12 month Self-Coaching program, to:

- **identify your Master Game**
- **live your Life Purpose**
- **enjoy a Fulfilling Love Life**
- **raise Positive Kids**
- **enjoy Vitality, Virility & Longevity**
- **have Financial Abundance**
- **develop an Impeccable Character**
- **have More Fun**
- **enjoy More Recreational Activities**
- **create an Energizing Work & Home Environment**
- **and more**

Just imagine this …

What if … Your past didn't matter?

What if … You had a *second chance?*

What if … Tomorrow began with a clean slate?

What if … You could neither fail nor lose?

Why not … Enthusiastically create and step into **Your 2nd Life** now?

♥

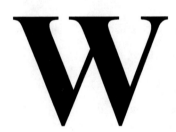

HEN A MAN REALLY LOVES A WOMAN
Why We Must Love More
And What To Do About It

by Colin Hillstrom

THE SECRET OF A BLISSFUL LIFE

The essence of Life on Earth is LOVE.

Love is why we are all here -
to learn how to give it, unconditionally,
and to learn how to receive it, gracefully.

Mastering the lesson of real love is man's greatest challenge.

This task appears in front of every man in the form of woman. To rise up to this challenge it is vital to know that - while a man remains immature psychologically, he will fail again and again, at truly loving a woman.

An immature man, who is nothing but a boy in an adult body, will seek what all boys want: excitement. This excitement after puberty is the sex that immature men crave so much. But sex is not what a woman wants.

An adult male who is insufficiently integrated is too much boy and not enough man to really love a woman. Instead of giving love, he selfishly demands sex and attention, and he uses all sorts of tricks to satisfy wants, even to the point where he aggressively manipulates and violates people.

Man and woman are meant to be One.

We are sexual beings. Sexual energy is our life force. Being sexual is part of our divine nature. However all too often this sexual energy becomes caught in the lower levels of consciousness where the human ego / mind is immature and not yet fully integrated. When we use our sexual, life force energy selfishly, it depletes itself pre-maturely and we die of dis-ease and old-age before our time.

This is true for both men and women. The soul that yearns for love and union remains unfulfilled, and its sadness is felt as pain and suffering through our mind, body, emotions and spirit.

The union of man and woman through unconditional loving - both physical and non-physical - reconnects us with our essence and our source. A male who fails to become a whole loving man keeps himself and his mate in a downward spiral of fear, separation, loneliness, dread, doom and gloom, worry, shame and guilt.

How did you feel when you first fell in love? Were you on top of the world?

In a perfect world, that love should have lasted. Reality is different. What can you do about it now?

It's simple: forgive and forget, and acknowledge the love that flows through your life this very moment.

Instead of blaming your mother, your father, your lover, your priest, your teacher or your friends for what went wrong with your love life, just try this:

Commit to being even more loving from this moment onward. Soon you will enjoy blue skies again … your fortunes will improve and you will begin to spiral upward in your experience of love and life on Earth.

Any man can do this! Any woman can do this!

Noticing and cherishing the beauty in everything that you see, feel, hear, touch, taste and smell is the secret of a blissful life.

♥

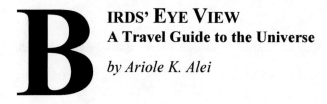

Enter Seclusion

…

The command. Like a directive. Gentle, yet affirming. "Take a bath."

I was becoming familiar with these 'directives'. Like firm requests. They always led to a discovery, even though initially each one, to my naïve mind, seemed initially odd.

"Take a bath."

I already knew how to discern. This is an ability which exists in all of us, albeit somewhat latent in many people. The ability to listen within, and to identify that which is benevolent and that which is malevolent. In seclusion, this ability was being rapidly honed.

So I knew, as with every one of the directives that I would ultimately receive from my guides, no matter how 'dangerous' they might appear, that I was truly safe in each and every one of them.

Discerning this, I entered the bathroom, and began to run water into the huge crowfoot tub. I stripped off my clothes, and I stepped in.

Some minutes passed ... and it didn't seem evident at all 'why' I was there. Me, water, the tub. Was I just ... to 'take a bath'?

I played for a few moments with a yellow plastic duck, truly at odds with the 'why' of this directive.

Then it began, as swift and clear as these experiences always were.

It was as if ... I was listening to ... a radio. And there was static. The ... wires were being ... tuned. And I was now hearing ... it was like a short wave radio station ... a transmission from ... *very far away.*

As this, and all of the phenomenal experiences which were 'delivered to me by my guides', was so effortless to me, I assumed that what I was hearing could be heard by everyone.

I listened. It was 'the news'. Just like an announcer, his voice piercing through the static, his message being heard. "The war is over."

And with that, the transmission ended.

I was 'released', from the bath. As its purpose was over.

I stood up, toweled off, and dressed, unsure precisely what it was that I had just heard.

I walked into the kitchen and, holding a glass of water in my hand, stood facing the window. When I began to hear it. It was *so loud.* Like New Year's Eve, and everyone leaning out of their windows, with noise makers and horns. *Celebrating!*

I assumed that it was all around me - in the 'world', outside. Then … I realized … I could *feel* it. 'Up' … 'above me'! *It was in the galaxies. It was our 'Festival of Friends'.* [1]

They were celebrating! Our freedom from the war! They were celebrating - the imminence of our coming Home!!

I felt them, my long forgotten 'spirit' friends. The thousands of spirits I'd left behind, when I 'incarnated' this time. They were still there. All of them (except those who'd incarnated, too). And they were greeting us. Jubilant that soon, 'Time' would be done. And the purpose of 'form' would be complete. And we would be united, again.

---

[1] Bruce Cockburn, a gifted and prophetic Canadian singer-songwriter, writes of our 'Festival of Friends'.

I assumed, in my innocence - for I had, all my life, believed that I am no different than any other, that we all have the same inherent gifts and abilities - that if I could hear this 'news', then everyone else on this planet Earth could hear it too.

I made my way to the living room, sure that I'd see striking changes in the world outside. There was no evidence of it. No evidence of the 'news'.

I called Ron, the last time I would speak with him. I cracked a joke! Something about 'the news', in 'code'! He didn't get it. *Ron* ... didn't get it.

And then I knew. If Ron didn't hear the news ... then who else did? Was I the only one? Or one of a very few?

Somewhat shocked by this, and feeling a tad alone, my guides slowly, ever so gently began to give me a sense of understanding.

They explained that, just like a star 'dying' and its light taking thousands of years to reach our sight, energy on other vibratory levels does this, too. Yes, the war *was over.* I had been led to hear this news. *It was true.* Yet it would take some 'Time' for the effects of this to reach the Earth.

I was, evidently, being attuned to what was taking place on the higher energy levels, 'ahead of our Time'.

This would be the first of several such 'prophecies' I would be shown.

...

The Return from the Quest

...

One evening there was a passion play in the theatre. The Conclave [2] organizers had known that I was a professional dancer. They asked me to perform the role of Lakshmi, as this was a passion play of the story of the gods.

One day in rehearsal, the cast was divided into two sections - the 'Light', and the 'Dark'. We were apparently going to enact the war.

The director arbitrarily drew a line down the centre of the rehearsal stage to make the division. I was, initially, in the cast of the dark. It felt so wrong to me. As we had been asked to bring black and white clothing for these particular costumes, and I had been guided to give away anything black, I simply said that I only had white clothing with me. This apparently sufficed. I was moved to the side of the 'Light'.

The staging was organized. We were given our cues. The 'Dark' was to physically oppress against the Light. And the Light ... was supposed to fight back.

My body froze. Not in a sense of shock, or fear. It froze in the sense of immobility. I had never received such a clear, easy to

---

[2] A Conclave is a secret spiritual gathering. This one was 'advertised', yet only those who recognized its significance would Know it and feel called to go.

discern physical message before. It was obvious. My body would not move.

I discretely removed myself from the rehearsal hall and made my way to my hotel room. I lay down on the bed, and I listened in. What was going on? What was I being taught? What was I being shown?

Light need not fight. Or justify itself. Truth is.

I wrote a note to the Director, explaining that I could not perform in that scene. I disclosed why, unattached to whether or not he would 'see' it, and understand.

♥

I entered one of the seminars - late, as I'd just come from a rehearsal. There was a man at the front of the hall, preparing to show a series of slides. This man, Dr. Frank Stranges, had apparently worked in the White House and had met the people whom he was describing. 'Aliens', he affectionately called them, with a knowing glimmer in his eyes. To be precise, Venusians. They had no body hair. Were supremely intelligent. And had offered to share with the US government technologies which would benevolently eradicate famine, war, and disease.

Apparently the government aides asked for time to consider this offer. They came back to the gentlemen and declined it, saying that it would 'disrupt the economy too much'.

Frank began to show the slides.

It wasn't that I recalled these particular men. It was that ... I recognized their *features*. The ... 'shape of their faces'. And more profoundly, their *essence energy*.

I had 'awoken' to the Venusians. I remembered them. As a 'race', as a species similar yet distinctly different from us - from humans.[3] And I saw in them, a key. For Pedro - whom I'd awakened to only weeks before - I now recognized. He ... was Venusian, too.

♥

Pedro.

My friend Mark, from the bookstore, suggested that we take a long weekend trip, rent a car, and drive to Mount Shasta. He'd been there. An amazing hike, he said. The air got thinner and thinner as you climbed. He'd never made it to the top. He felt it was time to try again.

We drove there, and camped. I began the ascent of the mountain with Mark, and felt a strong 'pull' to come down. Apparently, this wasn't why I came.

---

[3] Their civilizations are harmonious and highly intelligent models of planetary culture. They live an 'ethic' of benevolence, like an entire race full of compassionate Boddhisatvas. Theirs is a society of Joy, of Love, of Peace.

Venusians can't be 'seen' by standard human technology, as they exist on a higher vibrational frequency than we do.

Jesus is said to have been of Venusian 'origin'.

I discretely waited out the weekend, conscious that I didn't want to sour Mark's evident delight in his hiking.

Early on our last morning, we packed our gear into the car and began to drive home.

Mark was in the front seat. I had a strong, emphatic sense to sit in the back. The reason why would soon evidence itself. I needed privacy - quiet, no conversation - to experience another trance.

As we drove - 'away' from the magnitude of Mount Shasta - Pedro came almost forcibly into my mind. I had known 'of' him. A dear friend of mine had raved about a concert he had given in Vancouver not long before.

Why was he presenting himself to me? It was as if ... I was supposed to 'notice him'. As if ... there was some significant connection between us. A connection which was beginning to *wake up.*

This was all quite a mystery to me, still, as we returned to Vancouver. Mark dropped me off at the friend's apartment where I was staying. I found myself, once in the quiet of her home, gravitating to her stereo. There, atop a stack of CD's, was one of his. I put it on.

It was like I was an innocent child, suddenly plunged into maturity. I flew toward the speakers, hugging my ears into them *so*

tightly. I would have climbed inside, if I physically could have.
What? What was he *saying?*

He was talking about the eagle. Flying into the Light. Just
like with Alessandro's poetry which Shakey had decoded for me -
like his own recent 'First Folio' writings 'through' me - I could hear
the deeper meanings of Pedro's words *on their many levels.*

I knew too, with acceptance and a wave of resignation
throughout my entire being - like a mysterious sense of 'defeat' - that
Pedro, like Alessandro, might not know himself exactly 'what' he
was saying. Was he awake? If so, to what degree? Was I hearing
something 'through' him, through his words? Or did he know it,
too?

I was distinctly aware that I had no idea - 'why' I was
remembering Pedro. Other than to feel less alone knowing that he,
too, (at least on the level of consciousness of his lyrics) 'saw the
vision'. Was there something that we were to do? I listened in for
further guidance, and I was shown that, together, he and I would 're-
create the forgotten language'. The language which we all - *all
humans on this Earth* - had once spoken, yet had forgotten. An
ancient, unifying language *which we all would speak again.*
…

England Calls

…

I knew it was Time to go to England - London to be precise. It was Time to 'call' … the London Beak.

Many of the people on the conference calls were of the Beak. It turned out that, via connections - so and so knows so and so knows so and so - all of the Beak were, eventually, linked into someone in this group.

Yet it wasn't like sending out invitations. Because this was not to be a gathering 'on Earth'. It was to be a journey into deep trance, to awaken *collective memory*. And *only if the Time was precisely right* [4], would the 48 + 2 *know to come.*

I had personally heard several calls already in my life - 'calls' from the Higher Self, the unmanifest consciousness, the 'Great Soul' - to my 'little' self, my incarnate heart / body / mind. Jacob's Pillow, seclusion, the Earth Summit. I had followed these calls to places I'd never been, without research, completely through trust.

---

[4] In this mass awakening, each individual and the waves can only awaken to the degree that the *whole* will allow. Fear and unreadiness on anyone's part 'puts on the brakes', slowing the process down. For awakening has a powerful ripple effect. Each tiny degree of awakening consciousness effectively sets the entire mobile into motion, triggering - inviting, calling - the awakening, *the remembering,* of all Truth. For nothing is 'separate'. *All is interconnected.*

This critical principle allows us to grasp why Christ was crucified. Not all energy was ready. And so 'he', the vehicle, the catalyst for the ultimate awakening, was blocked from fulfilling his task - of awakening incarnate consciousness to its memory of itself *as the Light.* He and his life were designed to gradually - in the course of one lifetime - dissolve the *Veil* from the consciousness of 'men'. He was meant to 'lift the lid' - *so that we would fly free again.*

It has been two thousand years of 're-design' since then. And now … here is the 'Map'.

So if the London Beak Conclave was to take place now, I could only trust that my fellow souls of the Beak would hear this, their call, and follow it.

I gave away most of my belongings. I left the continent of my birth in this lifetime. And I flew.

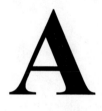

AWAKENING INSTINCT
The True Feminine Principle
by Ariole K. Alei

Introduction

There is a general malaise rampant in our culture, a malaise which threatens to destroy our very existence here in the 'world' of physical form. It is a malaise which arises within us - within our minds, the way we think and perceive of ourselves, the world, and what is beyond it.

This malaise can be seen as a loss. It can also be seen as a bloating.

Either way, the medicine for its healing - the elixir - is within us, within our capability. It is simple, yet not easy. To employ it is to call ourselves up from our depths. To employ it is to become the simple, unadorned, full potentiality of human.

The 'bloating' can be seen as this. We have, simply put, become grandiose in our thinking and have transferred numinosity from the divine to the mundane. In so doing we have cut ourselves off from instinct, the very signal that would redirect us to our sanity - and our survival / thrival.

…

The Numbing of Instinct

To understand how we allowed and participated in the numbing of our natural, internal 'signal' mechanism of instinct, we need to look at several historical elements.

Firstly, the relationship and interplay between the masculine and the feminine.

We have entangled our perception of the male and female with the masculine and the feminine. The latter two are principles, not genders. Each man has within him both principles, as does each woman. As a species we have come to overvalue one and undervalue the other, to our peril.

...

Awakening to Denial

To understand the numbing of instinct, we must understand denial.

Denial is the choice to be unconscious.

Why would we choose to be unconscious? We choose, at some level of our ego, of our mind, to be unconscious when we fear that we are unable to face what is - to respond holistically to what is. Denial can only exist in the presence of self doubt. If we believed in ourselves and had access (through our instinct and intuition and our heeding it) to all of our wisdom and personal, inner power, then we would have nothing to fear. Ever. We would be in an 'enlightened state of consciousness', something which I believe is attainable to each one of us, here and now.

...

Awakening our instinct and our intuition are the simple pearls within our oyster shells. Instinct and intuition naturally lead us out of the spell, out of denial.

...

Feminine Principles

I speak of instinct and intuition as feminine principles because they *require receptivity to be heard.* To develop one's relationship with one's instinct and intuition, one must be willing to learn how (and this is a very personal experience - no two of us are completely alike) to quiet the mind and still the activity enough to *be receptive.*

...

Your role is to allow them to arise.

Once the messages have arisen, there is a 'bridge' - a neutral bridge, neither feminine nor masculine - before the masculine principle is required. The masculine principle is the *action* in response to the intuition or instinct's message.

This 'bridge' is the teeter totter moment. It is the moment when either we take seriously, respect and honor, and commit to heed the message of the instinct / intuition, no matter the 'price' ... or it is the moment when we deny our inner wisdom and sacrifice ourself. In sacrificing ourself - our intuition / instinct - we are always sacrificing the health, the life of the system, too.

...

Always Benevolent

Intuition and instinct are always benevolent. They arise from a level of intelligence which is beyond - read 'incapable' - of manipulation or self service. They are always about serving the larger whole, the larger 'good'.

This is not to say that they don't - often - lead us to be catalysts in our own life and thus in the mobile(s) of which we are a part. By their very nature, they do shake things up.

Yet to understand - and to value this, without fear (in fact, dissolving fear) - we need to *discern* the distinction between destruction and deconstruction.

...

Being a Catalyst

When we heed - when we follow the 'advice', the leadership - of our instinct and our intuition, we are always, to greater and lesser degrees, called to be a catalyst. *We are called to be an agent of change.* This change may be 'lesser' in terms of effecting a minor swing of the mobile, evidenced mostly in our own life and in a seemingly minor way. Or this change may be 'greater' in terms of effecting us to the depth of our core, and/or effecting major change in one or several systems.

Intuition always leads to change. It leads to growth (not in an economic sense, as the word has been co-opted to mean). Though sometimes it does, through its liberating energy, lead to economic growth too! This is what is referred to as the 'bi-product' of prosperity. It is a secondary result of a primary, inner change.

♥

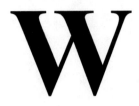# INDOWS THROUGH TIME
A 'Possible Evolution' Story

by Ariole K. Alei

...

When we and energy were sucked into this 'reality', we were split into duality at the point of departure from the fourth dimension. Again, imagine a water faucet. Within the pipeway and the faucet, the water is unison, together, one. As it exits from the faucet, compressed and channeled through a pathway and now exploding into 'open space', 'sparks' of water fly out in all directions. Power and fury, energy and chaos. What was once a harmonious cohesion of substance is now distinct and opposing droplets.

As we passed through the 'faucet' of the fourth dimensional portal, all energy was split in two and further divided. It was at this very gate that there came to be duality and polarity. It was here that matter and spirit became 'distilled' and separate. (The soul plane, to which disembodied souls 'rise' upon separation from their material bodies at death, is 'between' the earth plane and 'God', or the fourth dimension. The difference between 'death' and 'ascension' is that in death, the soul separates from the body, while in ascension, we take our bodies, which by then have shed all but the vibrations of *positive* energy, with us.) It was here that, not only was soul separated from body, even our souls were split in two. Hence, our awareness on various levels of the existence of 'soul mates'.

The opening to this pathway, or black hole, or 'umbilical cord' through which we came, is visible to us within this galaxy. It is the star An, the center star in Orion's belt. It is An where rests the 'focal point' of God, the star through which this universe inverses.

♥

When I met 'God' one thing startled and surprised me. First of all, I had never expected or even consciously desired to 'meet' God / Source / Creator / All. I wasn't even sure for myself that she/he existed or what, in 'reality', he/she was.

But it all seemed quite normal, in an odd sort of way, when I found myself kidnapped into seclusion to reconnect again with four of the nearest tiers of god energy.

What surprised me, as my four 'guides' came to be of clearer resolution, so to speak, ... and as each of them came to reveal clearly their own distinct energy and personality, ... was that 'God' seemed to me to be so sad.

This puzzled me as it confounded me. I had never been brought up with religious teachings and therefore had scant fluency in the way of religious notions let alone doctrines but ... Wasn't God the Almighty supposed to be an angry, totally in-control, ... man? I did experience god as 'male' in balance to my female energy, but ... the sadness. I asked Shakespeare's soul, another guide, "Why is God so sad?", for I was aware of a most forlorn, painful mourning and Shakespeare said, "Lille One[5]. You will know, in Time."

Months later, and my journey more familiar, it was all explained.

The personal healing which is taking place now for so many people around the world (- it is synchronicity rather than coincidence that like great sweeping tides our memories are being unlocked, revealing abuse of power and pain in many people's pasts, and *healing* it), this personal healing while one is walking through it may seem to be the most enormous flame that could exist. It is huge (though like the wake behind a boat, this path is becoming easier for those who follow in the paths of pioneers). And yet this 'horizontal' healing of our pasts and our long pasts (past lives) is simply a model of practice and experience for the 'vertical' healing - the healing of our relationship with 'God' and with our fuller selves. For as the 'film' dissolves and the veils of deception fall, pure god energy is beginning to reach us again. We are experiencing it in many ways,

---

[5] The name by which Shakespeare endearingly speaks to me. Meaning delicate one, innocent one, as if an elder speaking lovingly to a child.

finite now, and sweeping soon. The most obvious of these initial signals are the mass reconnection with our 'inner children' and our more deeply conscious selves, the 'horizontalling of hierarchy' and the return of accountability, our awakening to global crises and to the interconnection of all things, and the beckoning call to return anew to community, to cooperation, and to hope.

All of this is about trust. The challenge is about trust. Humankind in our state of limited memory has been deceived, abused and abandoned in ever-increasing ways. It has been many years and many lives. As the veils are lifted, and our trust anew is challenged, who will believe that the perpetrator was not God? Were we not taught that 'God' created good *and* evil? What if *this* very teaching were the lie?

Who would believe if 'god' were another being, equal to us and yet simply closer to multi-dimensionality, more whole and more 'alive'? *Will* humankind walk through the healing, our so-perceived 'gods' to reunite?

After all these years, it seems so far-fetched to be true.

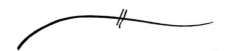

What do we have to lose?

A planet. Our species. And our life. For ever *and* all Time.

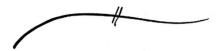

This … is God's sadness. Our Wills, to re-unite.

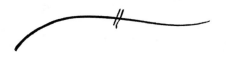

Whether or not we actually return to multi-dimensional existence is almost beside the point. The point is that we're dying. And if we're going to preserve ourselves in *some* form, 3D or otherwise, then there have got to be some major changes. Like One.

Orient ourselves towards the positive. Orient ourselves towards the positive. Orient ourselves towards the *Light*.

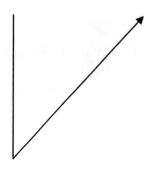

Shift, into the Light.

Going *Home.*

To focus on fear is to stay in the physical.
To focus on becoming *Love* is to fly free.

Home ... in to the *L i g h t*.[6]

---

[6] *Light* is beyond light and dark. A state of existence - a vibratory frequency - beyond the limitation of duality, it is re-accessed by us through our integration of shadow into light. This return to *Light* is the ultimate end of codependency, of carrying aspects of each other – projections and disassociations - us for them and them for us. It is the untangling of the 'web'.

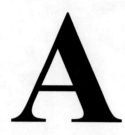# ASCENSION TEACHINGS
The Original Memory
* audio cassette series *

by Ariole K. Alei

From the Liner Notes
* Note that Dark and Grey refer to energy rather than to race or color

> *through the back door*
> *silently*
> *fold over*
> *to a new   breath*
> *of love   and light*
> *golden,   white light*
>
> *no struggle   no war   no confrontation*
>
> *just the gentle,   huge hands of*
> *love*
> *washing over the planet*
>
> *till all is Love*
>
> *and All is Light*
>
> *and Dark and Grey*
>
> *are no more*

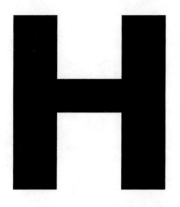

eartSong Matchmaking ™

... 'HeartSong Singles'

also HeartSong Couples, Families, and Teens

I, Ariole have always been a natural matchmaker. I love bringing together people, ideas, and environments to stimulate, inspire, and encourage us all to grow.

Even before we met, Colin had a dream - a vision - of creating a global 'spiritual matchmaking' service. A service dedicated to bringing more love onto this planet through teaching and supporting the evolution of healthy, respectful, soulful relationships. He saw this primarily as between male and female. As we all have both male and female aspects within us, we know this to mean also between woman and woman and between man and man.

We met as a result of Colin's search for a co-facilitator for his relationship workshops - someone to lead participants into their bodies through meditation and dance. He found me.

I also found him. That's a story. I had a vision ... and I followed it, to a tee. And there he was.

Within a year of our coming together we held our first Couples relationship workshop. It was so rich and delightful. Full of learning, joy and fun.

Yet I felt that I wasn't ready to be the co-facilitator and co-founder of a highly visible 'company' dedicated to bringing more love into this world through relationships. I had much more learning, and growing, to do myself first.

It is seven years later. And the container holds the space - and the magnet - for the growth within it. Our relationship has been my container. And Colin's love for me has been the magnet calling me out of my former wounds and fears into the strength and splendor of who I am now. And I, for him, have been the same.

Witnessing Colin's growth and evolution has been marvelous. This is one of the many gifts inherent within a soul-based relationship. We get first row seats in celebrating the intriguing journey of self-discovery of our mate.

HeartSong Matchmaking ™ is Born!

In April 2006 **HeartSong Matchmaking™** was birthed into this visible world. A 'child' of our parent company *Veraxis* **Coaching and Training™**, **HeartSong** is "the world's first holistic matchmaking service - designed specifically for personal growth oriented singles".

Members are *Lifetime Members.* We support our Members *holistically* in the four inter-connected life areas of Relationship, Wellness, Personal Leadership, and Success *for their lifetime.* We recognize that love and relationship are an evolution. They don't begin and end in the meeting of someone unique. They are a process, a journey. And we guide and support our Members through their many stages.

HeartSong Matchmaking™ is about Learning, Healing, and Growing. We assist our Members to learn how to be in healthy relationships. We assist our Members to heal the past so they don't carry it forward into future relationships. We assist our Members to grow as people, as partners, as lovers, as friends.

We also custom-design services for **Couples, Families,** and **Teens** through **HeartSong Couples, HeartSong Families,** and **HeartSong Teens** - so that everyone can access our wisdom, guidance, support, and resources, no matter what stage of life they are in.

Interested in knowing more about **HeartSong?** Visit

- *Veraxis* Coaching and Training ™ at **www.veraxis.net** to discover more about our holistic services
- **www.HeartSongMatchmaking.com** to learn about "the world's first holistic matchmaking service - designed specifically for personal growth oriented singles"
- **www.HeartSong-Couples.com**,
- **www.HeartSong-Families.com**, and
- **www.HeartSong-Teens.com** for further information on these specifically

E-mail us at **info@veraxis.net**

Call us at **604.731.1783**

It would be a pleasure to serve and support you!

May we create a planet of happy people, loving and loved, respectful and respecting. Imagine it. How would this world be different ... if there were more people in loving relationships, learning how to respect self, others, and this marvelous globe ...